Ex-Library: Friends of
Lake County Public Library

Awaken the DIET Within!

Julia Griggs Havey

Taking Control of Life!

LAKE COUNTY PUBLIC LIBRARY

**I invite you to go to my website at www.JuliaHavey.com —
and e-mail me a message, comment, question or any type of
communication. I try to respond to everyone.**

Or you may write to: **Julia Havey
P.O. Box 6794
St. Louis, MO 63122-6794**

**Cover photo: Suzy Gorman
Cover design: Tim Trunell**

3 3113 02014 8146

Copyright ©1998 by The Health and Wellness Inst.. All rights reserved. No
copying, distribution, or reprint of all or any portion of this book in any form,
may be done without written consent of The Health and Wellness Inst., and the
author of this book.

Always consult a physician before beginning any exercise or weight loss
program, or changes in your diet.

© 1998 The Health and Wellness Inst..
Printed by Scholin Brothers, St. Louis, Mo

Taking Control of Life!

INTRODUCTION

Thank you for purchasing my book, and congratulations on your decision to make positive changes in your life! I am confident that if you follow my easy-to-maintain guidelines, you will have success in your weight loss goals and positive personal development.

The basic principles behind this book are just that... basic principles. Too often we forget the basics, the basic rules necessary for healthy living, which allow us to build the foundation for a healthy, fulfilling life. It is for this reason that I have tried to keep this book from being lengthy, dull, and boring (hopefully!). I've described my personal story and given you simple principles for living a healthy, happy life.

My personal belief is that the diet industry and the variety of opinions it gives us, don't relate to our everyday real world lives. Few know what it is like to live life over-weight, like those of us making up the 76% of Americans with weight related issues do! Books by "experts" whom have never been overweight, tell us that THEY have the answer to what ails us! Or some celebrities claim they were once too fat to land a particular role, therefore they know how we feel and THEY too have the answers for us! Please! I have never seen overweight pictures of most of them! While all these books make for a good read, the programs were usually too complicated for me to follow and the foods rather elaborate for my culinary skills! There is a part of me that read these books with the skepticism of "sure, they are rich, they have chefs on call! If I could have someone cook for me, and a 24 hour personal trainer, I would loose weight, too!" And although I sometimes think this, I know how desperate I was to follow anyone's advice for losing weight. Therefore, I realize that there is some benefit in having a role model, and reading their books for encouragement. And as you will see, my story is what I hope for you, an encouraging one, that gives you insight of the pain caused by being overweight, and how a full and meaningful life is in front of you!

Let me say, though, if you don't truly desire to lose weight and make changes in your life, and you are content with all areas in your life, you will only get out of this book what you are putting into it. It is only those who deep inside feel they must change that eventually will get on the right road. As the title suggests, I believe you must look within for the strength and courage to get over the hump, and unlock your full potential as a happy, healthy being!

So if you are fed up with feeling as if your weight is taking over your life and controlling you, read on! The following story of the tragedy that I overcame in my life will help you reach into yourself to find the strength to improve your own physical, mental, and spiritual esteem- and therefore your overall beauty. It is most important that you discover your LIFE! And I hope that my message will help you with that discovery.

Julia

Taking Control of Life!

FORWARD

A forward by Dr. Bruce White, FACS

Throughout life it seems we're often looking for the easy answer to our problems, looking for the magic pill that will bring us wealth, or make us handsome or beautiful. Yet there are no magic pills— only the decisions we are faced with each and every day to work hard for the goals we wish to achieve. Weight reduction is no exception. It was so refreshing to meet Julia—she understood that weight reduction was a complex problem requiring a concerted effort to solve.

Regardless of one's metabolic rate or absolute weight, losing weight requires taking in fewer calories than one burns on a consistent basis. Unfortunately, diets concentrate only on the reduction of calories, ignoring the expenditure of calories. More importantly, they ignore the permanent changes in attitude and habits necessary to keep the weight off for a lifetime. Julia intuitively understood this and has not only made a commitment to losing weight, she has made it fun.

It is my pleasure to know Julia and contribute to this book. The basic principles involved are sound and, if followed, will lead to a lifetime of permanent weight loss. Read this book. It's fun, it's enjoyable, and it may even change your life forever!

Bruce A. White, MD, FACS

WEIGHT MANAGEMENT

A **forward** by Charlyn Marcusen, Ph.D.

As a researcher, practitioner, and instructor of behavior modification, fitness and nutrition for weight management programs over the past decade, I have seen many people loose significant amounts of weight. Unfortunately, only a small percentage of these successful 'dieters' maintain the weight lost for more than one year.

Weight management has never been more challenging. The American lifestyle, diet and culture, with it's 500 calorie breakfast muffins and super-sized foods will not support your effort to lose weight, or to keep it off. Many of our careers depend on hours at a desk, on a telephone, or in front of a computer monitor. Much of our recreation time is spent as a spectator. There are no indications that this trend will improve.

The guidelines outlined by Julia Griggs Havey are not a diet prescription, but rather a method of, and motivation for, creating a healthy lifestyle that will help you manage your weight throughout your life. Julia has demonstrated that your personal mind set, fitness program and eating style must fit your life and become personal habits to truly be successful.

Although there is no escape from sedentary work environments, high-calorie foods, giant portions or other food temptations, weight gain is not inevitable. By following these simple strategies, you can combat our "hostile" diet environment and create a unique healthy lifestyle, which supports lifelong weight management.

Charlyn Marcusen, Ph.D.
Associate Director
National Research Council for Health

Taking Control of Life!

ACKNOWLEDGMENTS

I would like to thank the many people that helped me get where I am today. Although many negative things motivated me to take charge of my life, there were many people along the way that made my life more pleasant. Dr. Bruce White, I am indebted to him for the touches that his masterful surgical skills performed after my weight loss. Dr. White helped me in many different ways, most of which was believing in me and this book. Ardy,   who took the time to show me the way to properly exercise. She taught me to love the results as well as the work. To all those who encourage me still as I strive towards ultimate fitness!

Suzy G., photographer extraordinare!! She can take a nothing face, and suddenly make it all seem worth...wait, that's Mary Tyler Moore! I couldn't have found a more talented photographer anywhere— thank you, thank you! And Darrin!

To two of the most wonderful miracles that God has given me, Taylor (9) and Clark (5). It was just the three of us for a long time and together we have all grown and learned a lot. Those tough years drew the three of us closer, and I thank God every day for both of you. I am proud of the people you are growing up to be and I love and cherish every minute of being your mother. You are great kids! I hope that living amongst my roller coaster life has given you the "thrill of the ride" and taught you not to fear taking your own chances- remembering you only have one life— do it right!

To Pat P.—wow! Your believe in my awes me! Thank you so much! I plan to live up to it!

To the Tims— all three! You all have helped me in many ways that I am truly grateful for. Although there are three of you, you have all been an important part of making everything work.

To my sisters, sorry for sitting on your Barbie car! Maybe now you two will be able to drum up interest for "the list"— try the Enquirer! Your love has always been one of the few consistencies in my life! I love you!

My dad, you haven't always approved of my methods, but you never quit believing in me. I haven't always made your faith in me easy. You are my hero and always will be. Three of the biggest lessons you taught me; 'to thine own self be true,' "illigitimis non carverundum," and 'don't be a quitter', have always stuck with me. I love you very much!

To my closest friends- Dana, Caryn, Betsy, Cathy, Nancy and Val. I realized as I wrote this book that being my friend could not have been an easy task. Still today you endure me year after year, fumble after fumble. Knowing all of you has given me more laughter, tears and security than most will ever know. Even though I will never, ever, ever again play True Colors with any of you!— I love you all dearly.

And most of all, to my biggest fan and motivator—my husband Patrick. Without you my life would be incomplete. Your zest for life has made Clark a sports loving, happy and secure little boy. Your intelligence is showing Taylor the value of the mind and the doors that it will open! Most importantly, you made us a family and brought prayer to meal time! Your belief in me and of my dreams, never allowing me to quit, has given flight to my wings. I never knew what being loved felt like before you showed me! You have taught me many things, most importantly the value of listening! I love you! Thanks for sharing your life with me and bringing me into your family. They have shown the kids and me such grace, kindness, and unconditional acceptance! Every woman should have the in-laws I have!!

Taking Control of Life!

Finally, I thank you the reader for hearing my story, and believing that I can make a difference in your life, and more importantly that *you can* make a difference in your life. I hope and pray that I am a strong, positive influence in your life, and that you will succeed in all you do! After reading my story, you will know that you are not alone in your struggles to lose weight, nor are you alone in your desire to change! I hope that I show you that the light at the end of the tunnel is closer than you think!

Thank you all!

Julia

Taking Control of Life!

CONTENTS

PART III
"The Second Chapter"

PART IV
Managing a Healthy Life!

The following is a "Guide" that I kept in my wallet and read periodically as a constant reinforcement of where I was headed. The small card this came on, stayed with me for 4 years! These are great words of wisdom!

Guide for Starting Over

May I have the courage to begin again—
may I be ready to overlook the
difficulties, to overcome the obstacles
and to stay open to the moment
as best I can.

May I be patient enough to know
it takes time to start over,
and wise enough to ask for help
from friends and family
when I need it.

As I look to the future,
may I reflect on the past
and remember the lessons
it's taught me.

And, Lord, may I always remember
to look to You
for strength and guidance.

*used with permission of Abbey Press

PART

I

Awakening My Diet Within!

DOOMSDAY!

It was a typical day, making breakfast for the kids and packing Taylor's lunch, hurrying to get everyone ready, so I could get to the office on time. I would drop Taylor at school, swing Clark to the babysitter's, cruise by the bread store to get my bran muffin and diet Pepsi® (I was on yet another diet!). Of course, my luck, traffic, well at least that gave me a few minutes more to listen to the jokes the morning dj's were saying and have some time alone!! Alone was something I was familiar with, even with two young children constantly clamoring for attention, one can feel awfully alone without a husband and father around to share it with! I had a husband, who worked long, hard hours, physically as a laborer, and the after work rituals often kept him out late. When he'd make it. home, they were usually already in bed. Good thing, it kept them from hearing us bicker about where he was after work. He is not a bad guy, just into that good-ol'-boy rut of nights out with the guys and making fun of his "prettiest-fat- lady-he's-ever-seen" wife. We were in love once. Coincidentally I was thin then, and we didn't have kids and money worries— you know, bigger responsibilities. At the time I ate my worries away, avoiding the pain of facing these responsibilities.

Off to work

I arrived at the office my customary 20 minutes late. After eating my breakfast and doing about 2 hours of work, I told my boss that I wasn't feeling well and thought I would take off for the rest of the day. Given that despite my deplorable work ethic, I was still his number #1 salesperson and he knew he couldn't control me, reluctantly he obliged and home I went. On my way home, I made my usual swing by Baskin Robbins for my dietary lunch- Espresso and Cream Lite Ice Cream (to die for!) and dove into it for the rest of the drive home. My spirits were lifted, my thoughts of needing to lose weight far away, after all, it was Lite, I wasn't cheating!! I was convinced that if I kept up the 'bran muffin, ice cream, and pasta with cheese' regime and made it 2 times a week to step aerobics, that with in no time I would be svelte again! My marriage would be better, we would have more time as a family, it was going to be Ward and June Cleaver perfect! I was tired of watching all the families at the park looking so happy, the dad's pushing the kids on the swings! It wasn't fair that my kids only had fat me sitting on the park bench watching them play. I wouldn't dare venture into those play structures, I could get stuck or someone might make a fat comment. No way! I knew that if only I could lose the weight, he would be proud to be seen with us, then we would be one of those happy and well dressed couples with the perfectly behaved children. I was convinced that this would happen for us tomorrow.

Once home, I fed and played with the kitten and watered the plants, and thought about what to make for dinner. The mailman arrived. "Oh good, something to do," I thought. I was feeling a bit bored. I looked through the mail, mainly a stack of late bills and coupons. A letter from the new NFL football team that recently moved to town. They were selling seat licenses for huge sums of money we couldn't afford. Luckily my husband's job was offering financing to anyone wishing to support the new team! My husband and his best friend pooled their money for season tickets. I remember thinking, "he will be so happy if he gets them! Hey, perhaps he'll ask me to a game, I love football. I will lose weight and buy a cute fall outfit, we will look wonderful together, just like the old days." I was even excited about the tickets now. Forget that we couldn't afford them, we would be a couple again! "Life is grand! I will get on a diet—as soon as I finish this pint of ice cream! In fact, I won't buy anymore until I have lost 75 lbs! I can almost picture me in my fall outfit now!"

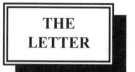

**THE
LETTER**

Finishing the stack of mail in front of me the last letter caught my attention. A letter for me? Hmm. No return address, wonder who I owe money to this time? Paying bills on time wasn't one of my strong points. In the moment that I opened this letter and read the very simply typed two sentences, my life was forever changed! It probably seems pretty clear to you already what that letter must have said, the clues were all there for me to see as well, but I guess I never wanted to put the pieces together! The words I read sent burning flashes through my body, I would have given anything to make it go away, but there they stayed, their message slapping me in the face as I read them over and over. "This couldn't be! There must be some mistake!" **What I read:** "Your husband is having an affair with Gina, it has been going on for over 2 years. Follow him next time he goes to Crestwood."

I had no idea what to do! Surely this was some cruel joke by someone who didn't like me!? He had promised me only weeks earlier that he would never have an affair the way our friend's husband had. He stressed that we would always be together! The baby was only 1! "How could he have been with someone for over 2 years?" It explained so much, and it hurt so bad, I didn't want to believe it was true. "He loved me, he called me everyday at work just to talk and say hi. Maybe he *wasn't* a family man— maybe he is just someone who likes hunting with his friends and hanging out having beer with them. Maybe I was wrong. I just don't know!" My thoughts raced in desperation with those questions. Flawed as he was, he was my husband. I thought it would all be ok— "its not true, it couldn't be! I wouldn't allow it to be! The kids and I need him!" Then I realized that I must still love him, why else would I be so upset. I thought of the good things about our relationship—

Taking Control of Life!

the funny jokes he would tell me, the trips we had taken. It dawned on me, all of that was in the past, very long ago, and there wasn't much about him or our relationship that was strong any longer. There wasn't much to convince me this wasn't true. I had no one of knowing for sure. Immediately, I knew it was time to fix what was wrong with me. "We will be happy again, I know it."

I paged him at the job site, said it was an emergency— after all, it was my rug that had been yanked out from under me and he had to set it right— I couldn't deal with this. I needed to hear him say it would be ok. What a relief, he was mad as hell, "someone is trying to hurt us!" He had no idea what this letter was talking about! Still, I was so upset that I headed up to 7-11® and got a diet Pepsi and cigarettes. I hadn't smoked in years, but it felt like the ideal time to start again. I couldn't stop crying hysterically. He said it wasn't true, but it didn't help. The truth was I didn't like myself then, and I sure didn't like the circumstance I was now in.

I called my best friend Dana, like the rock of Gibraltar that she has been for me for over 15 years, within moments, she was at my side to help me through yet another crisis situation in my life. Dana has a way of making a hurricane seem mild; she has her mother's wisdom and her dad's patience. She had no doubt that the letter was in fact the truth. However painful, it was better to know and face up to it and use the situation as a chance to change all that had been so wrong for too long. She was in some ways glad that this had happened. She knew how unhappy I had been for years. She shared the opinion of all my other girl friends. They all thought the reason that I over-ate was to hide from the problems in my marriage. I had two small children and didn't want to raise them "alone" and the Julia they knew would have dumped him long ago. Not one of my friends had any respect for my husband any longer. They had witnessed years of me showing up at couples' parties without him, enough to convince them that he was not the one for me. Little did they know, it was all I felt I deserved. After all, I was fat.

The Julia I had become was scared of divorce. I was frightened that I would become another one of the statistics— an overweight woman, left for a thin younger woman, left to live with little to no money to raise the kids. Hardly any women are better off financially after a divorce, usually resorting to selling your home then scraping by. I thought: "I love this house! I helped earn the money to buy it and make payments on it. It is the only home the kids know!" I didn't want to do that to the kids. I wanted them to have the perfect suburban childhood. I had convinced myself that an absentee dad is better than none at all. At least we had money to go to the movies and have the extras in life. "Who will want to date me?" I had been called a "fat" for so long, that I thought it was my *personality*, not a *condition*. I saw what lives divorced women I knew were living. I played up the fact I was married. Didn't that construe that I was also happy? What would they say to me now? I could hear the "I told you so"s coming!

I came from a divorced family, but I really didn't want to admit to the world much less to myself that I had made a mistake by succumbing to divorce. Who was I kidding, everyone believed that I had made a bad one from the day of my wedding. The questions about our decision to marry I wanted to prove wrong. I couldn't admit that I made a mistake, it was too late. "I would change him, I would make him a well mannered man, like my dad," I thought at the time. "Everyone would see I had found a diamond in the rough, I would be the Henry Higgins to his Eliza." I was the fool that tried to keep up the facade of the perfect family— I fooled no one. Obviously, that plan didn't work out.

When he arrived home that evening I would like to say that I kept my composure, but that would be untrue. I

> **Is it salvageable?**

fell apart, begged him to stay, said I would be a better wife, I would lose weight, we would be happy. He laughed it all off and said there was no truth to any of it and he didn't even know a Gina. He buried his head in the sand. I, for the first time in a long time, pulled mine out!

Many people hear of my weight loss success and say, "you got divorced, that is why you lost the weight." It may be summed up that easy, but the start of my weight loss was to try and save the marriage. It is important to note that the fear of ending my marriage was a big stick motivating me, although not everything can be saved if you wait too long, as you will see. It is important to note that when it comes to making some major changes in our lives, we do need a big stick to motivate us, as well as a big carrot!

I signed us up to attend our church's marriage counseling. It was one of the first phone calls I made— he refused to go. I soon found a counselor and his wife who help couples rebuild their marriage. They were wonderful. I started going in the hopes it would help us have a close and loving marriage, like we never really had, but one I had always wanted. He reluctantly went, as he made a promise to his mother. Keep in mind, he denied that there was another woman at this point. I was the "crazy lunatic" who just wouldn't drop it.

The counselor said, not discussing the affair was like having an invisible elephant in the room, we all know it is there and maneuver around it, but there it stays. He refused to acknowledge that there was an affair, he at best said he had a friend who was a woman, but that she was "older and overweight," that her 'ex' had been mean to her and her childhood was full of trauma, so he felt sorry for her. He said he wanted to give her a big bear hug. He had me feeling sorry for her. He insisted that she was nothing for me to be jealous of. So I continued the scheduled appointments, discovering things about myself I either never knew or long since buried away. Each week I felt stronger and more secure with who I was, and interestingly enough, I was losing weight, too.

I would recommend seeking counseling for anyone experiencing changes in their life. It is not a weakness or sign of mental illness to talk to a counselor, it is a great learning experience— about yourself! I am sure that had I not gotten counseling that I would not be where I am today. That is not to say you can't arrive at the same place on your own. I was feeling so low and so unworthy that having an unbiased ear to help make sense out of my life really helped me to discover me!

Eventually the truth came out, not from my husband- to this day he has never admitted to me that he had an affair or ever said that he was sorry. In a heated talk he will actually say to me, "you're not the first woman to get divorced," as though that makes all that he put me through acceptable since he didn't invent the concept of adultery.

Searching for truth

The identity of the "other woman" came to me in a dream. In the middle of the night, I sat up in bed and just knew that it had to be the woman whom he dealt with during his coffee business. I remembered that he had told me about a woman with whom he worked at this side business. "Why hadn't I put two and two together before now?" I thought. I confronted him with my realization, only to have him vehemently deny my charges, while asking me what I was going to do. I called his bluff and made some calls to ask if a woman named Gina handled the coffee vendors. "Yes" was the answer.

Woman's intuition was working for me. I couldn't believe that this woman was able to wine and dine my then husband at the most expensive restaurants in town and her company footed the bill. This discovery raised my energy level, and probably more my curiosity at the time, although it was painful. But even though we all have an innate desire for the truth, I didn't want to believe it. Denial is a great tool we use to avoid the truth.

I plotted some imaginary means of getting even. I came up with ideas that I thought would make me feel better—

Getting even?

adultery victims could use some constructive avenues to vent their anger. My two favorites were: "the Scarlet letter A cookie bouquet." Chocolate chip cookies in a long stem rose box delivered by singing telegram with lyrics revealing what was going on to the whole office. The other, having a huge Scarlet A set up in the front yard— instead of the hugely popular "it's a girl/boy" banner on a stork cut out, this would be an "A" with a banner that could read, "Adulterer." I know you're thinking I had way too much time on my hands to come up with these ideas, but I was in a state of anger and not thinking completely rational. I longed for the colonial America days where an adulterous woman would be publicly outcast and forced to wear the Scarlet A on her clothes, forewarning everyone of her sneaky and sinning nature. Acting on these would have been fun, and probably would have made me feel better, but I knew I would never stoop to that level. This, of course, was an emotional time.

The clever investigator

He went out that night for his routine "Friday-night-golfing-with-the-boys," leaving me and the kids alone. I cleverly came up with the idea that I could call the cable company to get information on this woman. So I made the call, gave her name (she has a unique last name and there were none in the phone book), and asked if they were my provider (as if I were her). They asked if I lived at ____. I said, "you bet" and I thanked them for the great service! I hung up and sped over there, thinking all the way the address they gave sounded strangely familiar. You guessed it, his truck was there. I banged on the door, but no one answered. I walked around back only to find the set of weights that I had bought him for Christmas lying in her driveway. He had said shortly after getting them, that he was moving them to his buddy's house so that they could work out together. In order to avoid self incrimination and destruction of property charges, I will stop here as to what happened to the weights and his truck. One note though, did you know that a 10 lb weight makes one heck of a frisbee? *It's amazing the strength you really do possess when the right emotion is present.*

I waited up for him, and at 4:00 am he finally stumbled in I asked him how the game was, and he said it was great. I asked him what his car was doing at Jeanna's house (he told the truth early on, he did not know a *Gina*, her name is *Jeanna!*). His only response was: "See, I knew we'd never make it." After being caught there, he still made it my fault. The fact that I caught him and was now screaming out of control at him was the problem as he saw it, not the fact that he was lying or having an affair. I cried and said that I was sorry. For what I am unsure, he hadn't noticed the damage to his truck. Still, I begged him to stay with me and give me that chance to be a better wife.

I actually still tried to re-ignite the long dead fire for a bit longer. I remember trying the candle-light, soft music, and champaign seduction scene— that was a bomb. I wanted to make it happen because I associated being someone's wife as part of being successful in life (which is being in a *loving* relationship is, as you will read later). My self-esteem was very low at this point, and without a husband I didn't think there would be a "me."

Why didn't someone just slap me. On my birthday, my parents took the kids and I to brunch. He said he didn't want to go, because he couldn't face my family. I didn't force him to go, I knew he was as embarrassed as I was over the whole mess. Through my counseling, I realized that I forced him to do things my way and be what he wasn't, far too often and for far too long. It's no wonder he went looking for a place where he could be himself. If we were going to make this work, it had to be a mutually respectful relationship and I had to start with myself.

As I was learning, you can only change yourself, not others. As you change, and strive to be the best person that you can be, only then can you positively impact the world around you. That is a lot different than trying to change what's around you not thinking that the problem is within you. "Was I actually growing and maturing!?" Self discovery is a wonderful thing!

After brunch, the old me drove by her house. He was in his truck in her driveway, obviously saying goodbye. I remember my first glimpse of her like it was yesterday— she had a red t-shirt on and white shorts. I remember thinking "white..before Memorial Day?.. how tacky! Obviously she has no breeding or class!" A hold over concept from my southern belle upbringing. I thought to myself, "I will definitely win him over this girl!" I guess I still had some confidence in me! Nice to know I hadn't lost everything that made me who I used to be!

Taking Control of Life!

I was also understanding the reason that he had the affair wasn't merely because I was fat or homely. It was that we weren't compatible. Most men stray probably most often for a younger feminine woman, while mine left for what I saw to be a woman who is more the outdoors-type—someone compatible. Hind site being what it is, I should have seen it all so clearly then.

Accepting fate

They were made for each other. I guess I didn't fit into his world, and looking back, *he into mine*. He once took me to a wedding in a small town where one of his work friends had a daughter getting married. Taylor was 6 months old and we took her with us, and you would have thought we were a perfect family to look at us. At that point we hadn't yet deteriorated, but things weren't great either. Looking back, even then we were the "Green Acres" couple in real life, if there ever has been one. I kept using the pay phone at the Elk's Lodge to call a client, leaving Taylor on her dad's lap. I was helping this client 'close' a deal and needed to stay on top of things. I have to say he *was* supportive of my career.

The women there looked at me like I had horns on my head— making a man actually feed his baby! My husband laughed and said his friends called me a city girl and said they should take me down to the river and dunk me to teach me a lesson. His dream life was to live on a farm and hunt and fish his days away. Not that there is anything wrong with that, it just isn't for me. I really had more thoughts involving dinner at nice restaurants, plays, parties with close friends, and great conversation. And even having my fantasy night of going to the symphony with a man who looked like he just walked off the pages of GQ!

I always imagined that I would marry a sophisticated

man— smart, handsome and entertaining. Things didn't quite work out the way I planned. It is said that people don't plan to fail, they fail to plan. I was happy with feeling as though I was loved, instead of finding someone that I knew I would love and be happy with.

We were as different as night and day. Perhaps each of us wished we had the qualities we saw in the other and maybe that is what drew us to each other in the first place. Who knows, or maybe it was the opposites-attract theory in action. Quite possibly I was just too immature to make a life-long decision when at that point in my life, my biggest decision had been what outfit to wear to a date or party. Even for decisions that simple, I surveyed for group consensus. Obviously I didn't have much faith in my own judgement back then. As they say, youth is wasted on the young!

As time went by, those who had known of the affair slowly came forward, giving me more pieces of the puzzle. It was like a drug, each time I heard some, I wanted to know more about this mystery woman. I wondered what her house looked like— was it more welcoming to a man than how I had decorated my home? Strange what details you focus on to distract your mind away from the important issues. Imagine my surprise the night when I found out I already knew what her house looked like. In fact, quite well because I had been in it numerous times in the past. No wonder the address seemed familiar to me— the house used to belong to one of our groomsmen and his wife! I felt like such a fool. I felt humiliated— poor, fat Julia, everyone feeling sorry for me behind my back.

That was perhaps the worst of the feelings I experienced throughout this ordeal. You learn who your true friends are. So many people knew for so long and no one cared enough about me to tell me... no one. I felt very alone, without a friend in the world. His "buddies" that would come over for dinner, hear him verbally bash me to them, knowing he didn't love me anymore, never once told me the truth. They would lie for him to their dying breath. To this day I do not know who sent me the anonymous letter. I suspect it was the "other" woman, tired of sharing her man and wanting him with her full time. Wouldn't that be something, her tired of sharing— I unknowingly shared him for 2½ years!

The final straw

The final straw came the morning our son had a 103 temperature. I took the day off work to stay with him. My then husband left at his usual 5:30 am time to arrive at his 8:00 am job. The wife of one of his coworkers, risking her husband's rage, had called me and told me she was so glad I finally knew and how the situation made her so angry. She told me more details of the affair than I probably needed to hear, and her words cut like a dagger through my heart. She told of him going over to this woman's house every morning very early before work, eating breakfast and getting a lunch packed by her. She said that since I started getting up early with him and making his lunch (my feeble attempt at winning him back!), that he would get to the job site and give the lunch I made away. She told of deer hunting trips that the mistress accompanied him on, even to the state reserve that my father got him a pass for. She told me the dog I reluctantly agreed to dog sit on one such trip was actually her dog and how the guys had a good laugh about that one. His only response to these allegations was to call the woman crazy for saying such lies.

The "gig" is up!

Rehashing the comments made to me by the wife compelled me to drive by the love shack on the way to get the Tylenol® for my son that day. I don't know why, but I had to go there. I couldn't stop myself, my heart pounding faster as I turned each corner. I don't have to tell you who was there. I drove, literally, into her front yard, screamed vile things about her as I got out of the car. At the top of my lungs I shouted his name and threw things at the house. Behavior I am not proud of, but I did it none the less. Eventually out sulked the adulterer, carrying his work boots in his hand and his cheating tail between his legs. The gig was up! He had been caught red handed by the "lunatic." He couldn't lie his way out of it this time. Although, to him I was the one in the wrong for daring to follow him there!

That was the final day of my "marriage"— my doomsday as well as the day of my awakening. I was no longer willing to subject myself to that kind of humiliation. The pain and the release that I experienced that day was like nothing I have ever lived through before. I was scared, yet exhilarated, mad, yet relieved. I was even about 40 lbs. thinner by then and knew that with time, I could get my life back in order— for me and for my children. Nothing I have ever done felt better than throwing all of his belongings on the front porch. As his things were being tossed out of the house, he said he loved us and didn't want to leave. He didn't have the decency even then to tell me the truth. I guess no matter how bad things get, there are some things that you just don't want to say for fear of hurting someone (me) who was obviously already in pain. But he certainly didn't want a marriage, either. At least not one like I had grown up dreaming of having or knowing would be right. I think he was afraid of what I would do to him, not what would become of the family we once had and now never would again.

I wasn't the most rational person those days and I suppose I was a "lunatic" at times. I would imagine so, because for over 2 years, I was called a prison warden for daring to ask where he had been. On nights when he would stumble in at early morning hours, I would ask his whereabouts only to be told "I am not going to stay home with you!" I felt as if 2 1/2 years of my life had been wasted. I could have been trying to rebuild my life long before it was the pathetic ruin I found it in now. My self-esteem had been torn down bit by bit, my heart ripped out a little more each day. My thighs grew bigger and bigger out of my eating for companionship.

Now, I was gaining confidence each day and with that came rationality. I have never looked back on that day with regret. I knew that no matter how hard it was, I would survive. I had known for too long now of his lies. No more. No more tearing each other down. I was free. We both were free. In many ways, I was glad for him. Had we stayed together any longer there might not have been any pieces of either of us left to pick up. I assure you that as much as he tore me down, I did the same to him in return. It became a insult fest when we were together. It felt good to just be away from it. I had a renewed sense of confidence and I was excited about getting back to living a worth-while existence.

Why?...Why?... That was my awakening. My rock bottom. Your story may be similar, or if you're luckier your spouse hasn't quit loving you because of your weight. I thought back with uncertainty— "should he have loved me less if I had lost a limb, or was disfigured some other way?" Fat on my body made him look away from my heart— it just wasn't right. I felt unlovable. "Why did he quit loving me? Why did I let *me* quit loving me? Why did I let this go on so long? Why did I make this decision? Why would anyone be like this? Why...?"

Perhaps my story will spark you to action before something sacred in your life is lost, as it was in mine. As I write of that painful period in my life, I do it knowing that there are so many others out there tolerating less than respectful treatment from others and from themselves, because they lack self-esteem, as I did. Think of the things you may have already lost that you can still get back— your health? you energy? your confidence?

I often ask myself, was it the fact that I no longer respected myself that those around me treated me the way they did? Or was their treatment the reason why I quit caring. I still don't have the answer, I think it is at best a combination of all factors. Either way, the same issue needed to be fixed—me! I needed to get back into the game of life and live it to the fullest! I needed to start looking within for the strength and power to change.

If what happened to me can teach you one lesson, I hope that it would be not to let food consume you to the point where you quit cherishing all of the gifts that life has for you! Your new motto should be— "consume food, but don't let it consume you!" I don't know if my marriage could have been a happy one forever if I had not gotten fat, if we would have grown together rather than apart. I will never know. I do not regret the road that I have taken because in so many ways it has made me a better person, but I learned that I will never take life, myself or those I love for granted ever again! I have also learned that being overweight has many more negative effects in your life than just ruining your health. It robs you of a full and rewarding life!

LIFE BEFORE

My obsession with my weight and body image began long before I became heavy. In fact, I had spent most of my 30-plus years obsessed with my body. Throughout my life, I'd find myself thinking, "I'm too fat; my thighs are too big; my chest is too small." I measured my self-worth by how others viewed my body and treated me. I sought my self-esteem via others' image of me, rather than MY image of myself— spiritually, emotionally...me, the person inside that really mattered!

One large infant! My father enjoys telling the story of my first brush with over-eating. After I was born my mother required a few more days in the hospital to recoup from an infection. Since dad had managed to raise two other babies without incident, they felt it was safe to send me home with just him. He marveled in his skill at caring for me! I was a perfect baby, for a girl; he was 0-3 at attempts for a son! Beautiful, healthy and could I eat! I was certainly thriving, my weight had nearly doubled in the week following my birth! It wasn't until my mother arrived home and pointed out to him that one must dilute baby formula that he realized I was merely bloated and about to explode!

As a child, I don't remember ever concerning myself with nutrition or healthy foods. My mother was a great cook and we always had good meals, we had to eat all of it, no mater how full you might be. I remember the cream filled tasty treats we would get after dinner while we watched Disney® on TV. There was always some wonderful confection around, either she was preparing for a bridge party or teaching someone how to make her gourmet treats. While my dad was in Viet Nam, I even got to get up in the middle of the night and eat ice cream with my mom as she watched the news for word of the war. How lucky I was, how loved,.. how well fed. They used to call me the 'dumple,' a pudgy lil' dumpling for short, I guess! I wasn't a particularly fat kid; not a skinny one either. Regardless of size, I remember other kids teasing me and calling me 'Griggs Pigs'. I vividly remember being crushed when a sales lady announced that I couldn't fit into a size 6X any longer. That moment might be what triggered my size obsession. A 6-X was tiny, petite, cute 'kid clothes'! I didn't want to wear the plus size "fat" big kid clothes. I think I just didn't want to grow. Continue to grow, I did, and children can be so cruel, I doubt that any of them realized how badly their school yard pranks hurt. It seems to just be human nature to make fun of people that are different!

My friends and I soon discovered my mother's stash of pre-made desserts that she hid in the freezer in the carport before big parties she was throwing. Who

Sneaking food

would ever miss a few—-dozen, that is! I doubt I will ever forget my mothers reaction when she in fact did find them missing! She took a turkey out of the freezer and threw it outside— goodbye Thanksgiving! Everyone was mad at me for ruining the holiday!

Now that my food source had been cut off, I soon began sneaking to the store on my bike to buy pop tarts with my friends and gorging on them before we would get home. That was probably the beginning of my unhealthy eating habits. I was a self-taught closet eater. It was the family mystery— how did Julia keep getting bigger? My parents really did try to set good examples. I was the only one to have a weight problem in the family! Like Homer (Simpson!) said..., "why do I have such a weakness for snack treats, doooh!"

As a kid we moved every year or so, because my dad was in the Air Force. The last military base we lived, was in Illinois. From my perspective, it was the worst! The "townees" were the snobbiest group of girls I have ever met in my life! Why still remains a mystery to me, but they didn't like me. My sister's theory on why the local girls always made our lives hell is that our dad was always one of the top ranking officers most places we went (even those who outranked him could never out shine him- dad is a flamboyant man!). I suppose we may have appeared attractive and well dressed, and noticed by the boys. I guess the girls felt threatened that the 'Griggs girls' would steal their boyfriends.

Adjusting

Back then, I didn't want their boyfriends, only their pastries! Besides, I had enough to deal with- I was 13, my parents were divorcing and my sisters were going off to college! For a while, it was just my dad, Nana and myself. Talk about bad eating habits! It was either the outrageously good, though very fattening, southern fried soul food my nana's helper made us, or my dad's "roast in a bag" special —I stuck with the pop tarts! That's when I developed my habit for skipping meals and only eating sweets. Dad did the best he could, he focused on the important stuff— making sure that I was happy and well adjusted! He spent time with me, although not cooking! They are my best childhood memories.

Riding horses with my dad was the most fun I ever remember having. He even crawled around ringing cowbells and making Phantom of the Opera noises to scare my friends and me at sleep-overs! He would show up for the mother/daughter fashion shows at my school or for the teas. He was great! His only big fumble came when I got my period. He just couldn't have "the talk" with me. He opted for giving me a copy of a "The Little Sperm That Could" cartoon book and telling me to call my sister if I had any more questions. You should have seen it, a suave little sperm in a top hat swimming up stream to try to be the first to meet the shapely egg perched on the chaise lounge ever so seductively. *It is one of my funniest memories.*

The next few years were quite an adjustment, I was a full-fledged obnoxious teenager and had a full plate (literally and figuratively!). Between caring for the horse that my Nana Mary bought me, my dates, dad's dates, keeping my sisters updated as to who was trying to land dad this time, I was busy. That is a novel waiting to be written. He was after all, the most eligible bachelor in the area and so adorable, the women wouldn't leave him alone. It was better than a Three Stooges film when I would see my sister move one particular woman's pots and pans out of our house every time the woman left them there. She kept trying to move in, my sister kept moving her out! I have always thought my dad was the greatest. I was right then and still hold firm to my image of him! (I hope he realizes I thought that, even while I was putting him through the hell of raising me!) He managed to find the right woman for him amidst the sea of prospects, they married and we began our new lives. He retired and we moved across the river to St. Louis.

Finally, I thought I would have a permanent home—friends that I could get to know well, and not have to say goodbye to anymore. A school where I could get to be part of the cliques, no more of these schools by the base where the locals have all known each other their whole lives and aren't about to let military brats into their circles! I was really looking forward to this!

Making friends

My weight wasn't bad, I felt like a normal (my parents might disagree!) teenage girl, I wore a size 10 or 12, and by my definition I wasn't fat or even chubby. Things went well for me at my new school. I had a boyfriend the first year there. I think my sister's theory was right after all because he was my only friend for quite a while. That is until spring when I met Dana, we were both playing the role of the devoted girlfriend, watching our guys practice baseball. We immediately became inseparable. Then, I met these other crazy girls in my Spanish class, immediately it spelled trouble. Little did any of us know what was ahead! With in no time we were known as the Big 8— eight girls, one crazier than the next!

The next few years of my life were the happiest I had ever known. I had a close group of girlfriends and we did everything together. I felt as though I belonged for the first time in my life. I even got a nick name for the first time, I was Jules (jewels)! We were a force to be reckoned with— we were cheerleaders or poms, we had the best parties, slumber parties, cake fights and more! We all shared the same appetites as well, and we could easily evacuate a refrigerator after school, sometimes without the formality of silverware!

Life isn't fair

As the world can be an unfair place, they never seemed to gain weight. That appeared to be my job. We dated the most popular boys. I usually dated guys from a nearby all-boys school, maybe they were more desperate than our guys who never asked me out, always preferring my friends! We thought then (and still do!) that we were the coolest. A few boys at school were such jerks to me, even though I was relatively thin (what I thought) at the time, they called me 'Namu the killer whale' and 'Buffalo butt'! How bullies are able to determine your weak point and then exploit it is beyond me, but there are those that are so good at it, they make it an art form. Mark and Bill were two of the best! They made my days torture! Mark even wrote of his nickname for me in the yearbook for all to see!

A girl with high self-esteem would have realized that these pimple-faced boys were merely looking for attention from one in the more popular group. It took the wisdom of a grown woman to reconcile that one! As a young girl it drove me to the Diet Center for an entire summer, slimming down to a practically anorexic 110 lbs.— at 5'8", that's a bit extreme! (I saw Bill and his wife at our 10 year reunion, she was pregnant and very huge! I starved for weeks before the event and did manage to look ok. Bigger than I had been in high school but I had a great new dress on and felt good. (I often wonder if he dares call her buffalo butt!) My willpower was intense that summer, the girls and I all went to a Bob Seeger concert and I only drank my diet Pepsi with lime while they imbibed in a few (root?) beers! I got so thin that summer, that my boyfriend du jour's father bought a candy bar and made me eat it! I look back now, with that grown up wisdom and it is so clear that all of the stupid decisions I ever made were out of an attempt to gain acceptance. I wasn't secure with who I was. I needed to hear from others that they thought I was great, because I didn't think too highly of myself.

How well I remember the craziness of weight obsession in my teen years— the unhealthy diets, desperate thoughts and strange rationalizations, there is not a diet out there I haven't tried—even the tuna and cantaloupe diet for an entire summer. Once, years later, out of pure desperation, I offered a friend $500 *to drive me to a hospital emergency department entrance and have her chop off my rear end! Then take me into the emergency room. Sure, I'd be horribly scarred but, at least I'd be thinner! (You've never been that desperate?). Another time, a friend and I jogged to the all-night bakery and ate a dozen creme-filled doughnuts. I guess we figured we could eat as much as we wanted since we had jogged a few blocks! Let me tell you, getting back was a lot harder than getting there!*

I'm sure you'll believe that I once bought a "miracle weight-loss pants" from an ad in the back of a magazine. You know those ads— 'amazing!, drop 20 pounds and a dozen inches in 2 days!' Maybe you even purchased the pants as well! The ad promised inches off my waist by the very next morning! I waited weeks until my package arrived, eating all I could in the duration, assured that the svelte body I sought was "in the mail." The package arrived and I hurriedly ran upstairs with it, tearing it open along the way.

In preparation for the magical transformation, I ran back downstairs to get the vacuum cleaner, then back upstairs to pull on the "miracle" pants made of something that resembled a plastic trash bag! I attached them to the vacuum, as instructed and

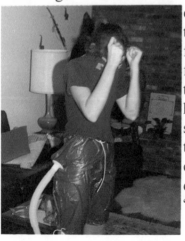

commenced running in place. I guess the idea was a "vacuuming-out of the fat on my body." Things went great for about 30 seconds. Then, in all of the excitement, the unthinkable happened. The rear end of the pants split wide open!! I was released from the compression seal, and thus, a complete 'blow out!' I was devastated! My dreams of a "playmate figure" were shattered!

Taking Control of Life!

As if was not humiliating enough, my sister wet her pants (literally) because she was laughing so hard! I went downstairs to find that everyone else in the house had heard the whole sit-com and they, too, were in stitches. I don't think they ever took any of my "dieting" seriously from that moment on. *I'm not sure I really needed it by looking at this photo!*

In college, I endured a pretty severe blow to my ego, and food seemed to ease the pain. That must be when I began to think that eating made things better. I dabbled with bulimia, it was the "in-thing" in my dorm. I wouldn't recommend that route for weight loss, it is very gross, leaves your eyes red and swollen, and can lead to severe consequences. I know of a few people who now, after 15 years, still dismiss my weight loss success by suggesting that I must merely be putting my finger down my throat. Sorry to disappoint them, this time I lost weight the right way, forever!

Difficulties in college

In my senior year of high school, all I talked about was becoming an ADPi—a sorority that my mother had been in college. She had also was the campus beauty queen, a teen Miss Florida—an Elizabeth Taylor double and an actual decedent of Spanish Royalty—for real! (We are related to the original first family of Florida, back to Ponce de Leon and all that conquistador history! The Count de Guemes or something like that! If America still used formal titles, I could claim my Countessa title as well!)

As a teen I used to fantasize about traveling to Spain and meeting my look- a-like relative and living amongst European royalty. It made living with those who snubbed me more bearable. I dreamed of the day they would all have to curtsy to me! I have a back issue of Town and Country in which my mother and my grandmother are posing outside Castile de Castellón in St. Augustine with the current Spanish Duke. I can't imagine he was too thrilled to meet his American non-regal relatives- if any of them were like me, that is! I wasn't there, but I know that had I been, I would have asked him if we had a castle or any spare tiaras he might not mind parting with! I can't imagine I am the only one who had such outrageous proposals for him! After all, we are family!

I didn't know my mother very well, I remember her as the outwardly perfect southern woman, very graceful and charming to others. I wanted to be part of her sorority. I felt that would somehow make us close. Growing up without her all those years, I wanted a tie to her. I never told anyone why it was so important to me, everyone thought I just wanted the social part, but to me it was more, a lot more. I would share something with my mother that was a huge part of her life. She went back to college after her divorce from my father and actually became a house mom for ADPi at FSU. Joining that sorority and being part of that group was all I wanted out of college!

Learning

My ignorance during those days stretched so far as to question my friend, Betsy, who knew that she wanted to become an engineer. I thought, 'why in the world would she want to operate a train?!' I was way too immature and unprepared to be on my own, much less in college! I had no clue what I wanted to be when I grew up, much less if I even wanted to grow up! My grades in high school were reflective of my 'don't-give-a-damn' attitude at the time, and therefore the sorority system that I so desperately wanted to be part of, turned it's nose up at me...ouch! They pushed my dreams aside with out so much as a chance to prove myself worthy! I had blown my chances without even knowing. If only my dad had told me why studying in high school was important, not the stuff about a career and grades, but about *sorority acceptance*, now that would have motivated me!! As they say, figure out why you want something and the how seems to take care of itself!

Oh well, I decided to take their advice, finally, and study hard this year and try again to join the sorority the next semester. It might have worked had I not discovered serious partying, fraternity guys and binge eating. I was too busy to study much. In keeping with my sisters theory about petty girls, it turns out one ADPi member really liked a guy I started dating that semester- like I knew?! Perhaps had they let me in their little club when I got to town, I would have known and would have steered clear of him! She 'blackballed' me on my next go-round and my hopes of ever being part of them were gone forever. The fact that one person has the power to deny another their dreams for such a personal jealousy didn't then and still doesn't seem fair to me! From then on, my college years went by in a blur of parties and dates, a few classes thrown in for appearances! Not to mention a few eating binges to ease the pain. The most serious diet I tried then was the "jog-to-the-all-night-bakery diet!"

I was miserable, I felt like everyone belonged to something except me. I really tried to fit in the college scene. I had all the right clothes and even my own car— usually an automatic popularity booster. However, it never seemed to work for me. I'd become very depressed and further into my disorders. I quit going to class entirely and confessed my desire to come home.

My dad insisted that I pull myself together, tell my professors I was sorry and would work hard to make up the work I had missed. Yeah, right! Like I had the confidence to walk up to a professor and admit errs...duh! That was the whole problem! I lacked any believe in myself or my abilities, academically or personally! I let one girl's blackballing of me eat me up inside! I felt like the biggest looser ever! I did manage to confront my philosophy teacher, he was 'cool' about it, perhaps he knew my karma was very low, he was kind of a "hippie!" He convinced me to stick with school and try. He would rank as one of those wonderful people whom I have been lucky enough to encounter along the way that really cared about me and tried to get me to see that I was more than what I gave myself credit for.

While home for Thanksgiving that year, our family's priest friend asked me how I liked college and what courses interested me most. Philosophy was my answer, as it was the only class I actually went to regularly. He asked if I had read the work of St. Tomas Aquinas, my face must have obviously drawn a blank stare of confusion on it. My father commenced grilling me as to who was St. Tomas Aquinas? Surely, I must know he insisted! Not to be humiliated, I gave it my best shot- I responded with certainty that he was, in fact, the founder of the Kiwanis Club. I thought it seemed logical. I don't know if their laughter was that of disbelief or shock— after all, we are Catholic and how could I not know the father of Catholic theology? I would forever remember him now!

After a few more years of the same, my dad eventually tired of my academic probation status and suggested I become a stewardess. I certainly had the credentials for that career! I loved to have fun and that was one fun job! It was also one of the few professions with weight requirements- my obsession continued! I had to be thin for my job!

Flying high! So I left school in hopes that change would do me good. I was accepted for the position, and the happiness that it gave me came out of acceptance- I belonged to an elite group! There was the weight requirement, though, and as time went on, I noticed (as did my boss), that I was always on the high end, literally, of the acceptable weight limit. Much like at the air force bases, when I was the bosses daughter, I caught a lot of flack at work. My dad ran the airport in St. Louis and this was the largest airline in the city. It was always: "she's *his* kid," or "wonder how *you* got the job?" So much for fitting in and being accepted. But, that didn't keep me from having a great time! I really loved the job and was good at it as well! To me, it was like hosting a dinner party every night- it was my job to make sure that every passenger not only got to their destination in comfort, but that they had a great time getting there! I was beginning to realize my strengths: I was social, not academic! I loved working first class on the long flights- TWA's service was very elaborate then. I made friends with a few of my coworkers and we had a lot of fun! A certain freedom came with being "his kid," although I tended to push the limits of tolerance of my superiors. What can I say, there is nothing like a whip cream fight in the lower galley on an L-1011(not that *I* ever did that!).

The lay-overs as a stewardess (of course, 'flight attendant' now) were a blast— site seeing in different cities and a lot of social activities, exactly what you hear of! One such lay-over in Hawaii coupled with too much sun, made for a very long flight home! I remember passengers feeling so sorry for my sunburned and blistered legs that they took out their aloe and rubbed me down. My more professional crew members didn't enjoy my style. I felt they may have thought I shouldn't be having fun because I was bordering the weight limit, and should take that seriously.

But the variety of restaurants across the country made for great eating as well! My years in college conditioned me for eating to feel good. *Too good* in my case, as I started filling out. Much to my embarrassment, and with a weight requirement, my male boss would have to weigh me... "Hop on the scale Miss Griggs."

If I was too heavy, I could be grounded or put on weight check. For years I struggled to control my eating and maintain my weight. Ex-Lax became a food group for me. I didn't think that I looked overweight back then. Recently I ran into a flight attendant I used to work with, she reminded me of the time I threatened to sit in a lounge chair at the security check point, wearing a bikini and hold up a sign reading "TWA thinks I am fat, do you?! Despite my climbing weight during my flying years I had a great social life! I met some very interesting people— professional athletes, lawyers, stockbrokers, real estate tycoons and even a wrestler— no Indian Chiefs though! I really believed that one day on a flight I would be discovered (for my crazy antics, I guess!) and success, fame and fortune would be mine!

I was lucky enough to meet many celebrities on board my flights, including Michael Jackson, Dan Ackroyd, Michael Keaton (he was so rude to me—all I did was ask him to introduce me to Elizabeth Taylor!) Audrey Meadows (she had to tell me "who" she was— "to the moon with me" she said!), Kim Basinger and more.

Without a doubt the nicest by far was Dan Ackroyd. As alcohol had become another 'pain killer' that I used in addition to food, I found many days where I experienced a hangover. It was he that made me a Bloody Mary (Virgin-to me anyway!) in the first-class galley to drink (I was very hung over!), the same recipe he and a 'old-friend John' used to have. He told me how he and Donna Dixon had said their wedding vows on a roof top- shouting down to the crowd! He was so great to meet, very down to earth and warm, except, that is, when I asked him if I could be in his next movie! He said, "you're funny kid, but you have to pay your dues, it doesn't happen easy for anyone!" I thought my big break was sitting before me. Little did I know how soon and for how long I would be paying my dues!

One night during the TWA strike, I met a union man who kept giving me a hard time about crossing the picket line and not supporting my union! He was handsome in a burly sort of way and I suggested he try to change my mind over dinner, laughing to my friends— "watch me fall for this one!" You guessed it— I married him, enough said about that already. We had a great time together, taking trips and having parties for our friends (you should have seen the two groups trying to mesh, it just didn't work!) My weight was creeping up then— I was about 160 lbs or so, compared to the 135 when I married.

About falling-in-love, I am not sure that was the case, hindsight being 20/20. I think even that

Falling in love?

decision was based on acceptance. He told me on our first date, that his "wife and his kids would always come first." I was not overweight then, and I wanted to be a beautiful bride. I wanted my dad, wearing his military mess dress to give me away. It all sounded like a dream to me, I would finally come first, be taken care of! He sold me on the destination, although the journey would be rather different. I wouldn't change it now because I am thankful to have the children, yet I often wonder "what was I thinking!?" I tell the kids that God must have some pretty important work for them to do while they are here on earth, if not, why would he have thought to put their dad and me together!?

To my relief, I became pregnant, just at the time TWA would have required me to lose 15 pounds. I now had a license to eat! I remember thinking, "Hey, I can gain all the weight I want now and you can't do a thing about it." Talk about cutting off your nose to spite your face— or in my case, stuff my face!

And stuff it I did! I was eating for two, wasn't I? Two pastries, two sundaes... I took full advantage of that situation! I wonder if any of my first class passengers noticed that their dessert offerings were skimpier on my flights than on others? Although I gained 65 pounds during my pregnancy, I didn't feel fat, I felt so amazing. I thought I was the cutest pregnant lady ever and dismissed the weight gain, convinced that the reason I had gotten so big was that the next NFL superstar was in my womb. I guess that I didn't realize that it isn't physically possible to 'carry' in the rear end—the biggest part on me! But anyway, alas (for my theory), I had a tiny baby girl— a six-pound, three-ounce baby girl! Hardly big enough to justify 65 lbs. of extra weight gain! So, along with my beautiful baby, I brought home 50-plus pounds from the hospital!

But never mind the fat, I basked in the joys of motherhood. I loved it! And since I was breast-feeding I, of course, needed extra nutrition to produce enough milk. Bring on the buffet! Needless to say, I wasn't one of those women who wear their pre-maternity clothes within weeks of delivery.

I gave up my flying career after accepting a buy out, an early retirement offer made by then owner, Carl Icahn. I was offered lifetime free travel— cool! They didn't have to ask me twice. I didn't return to my job as a stewardess. Good thing, I never could have squeezed myself into my uniform if I had to! I enjoyed my time off with Taylor (my newborn) and actually started to trim down. I had my 10 year reunion and starved until I could wear this great little red dress I bought! I loved being a stay-at-home mom. I could have done it forever if we could have afforded it. Instead, I entered a nine-to-five, sit-on-your-butt-all-day business world. My thighs and rear end thrived in this environment! I nibbled on snacks all day! My only exercise was walking to the snack machine—little wonder I kept getting bigger! I actually found my calling at this job. Sales! I found a job where my gift of gab didn't get me in trouble. It actually made me successful! *What great country we live in!*

Yet my loss of social life for being a mom and a "nine-to-fiver" limited my "party" life. Without alcohol,

> **Working 9-5**

food was all that was left as my crutch for feeling good. Through the years, I didn't know what I should be when I grew up and the answer had been obvious since I was a kid— sales. I am a born sales person. I've been told I can convince a blind man to buy roller skates (not that I ever would). As many would agree, I have the gift of gab. Now I was making more money than I could ever earn as a flight attendant and I get to be home with my little girl every night! My skills in life were clear, being social in my work! I really loved what I was doing for a living, it is a great feeling when you are not only good at something, but you love doing it as well!

The only problem for me was that a desk job was so sedentary. As a flight attendant, I was moving around the airplane all day and walking a lot in the cities I would stay in. I was never a jogger or exercise type of person, but at least I was moving. My life was a series of rushing to drop the baby at the sitter's, working all day in a sedentary job, and rushing to make dinner at night. It never even dawned on me to consider adding working out as part of my routine. My husband didn't get any exercise, it just wasn't part of our lifestyle and we went out to eat for our socializing. I gradually kept getting bigger— it happens so slowly that you hardly notice the pounds creeping up. It starts with a belt that is too tight here, an 'old' pair of jeans that you can't zip up there. The new clothes that I bought were more comfortable, so you move up a size or two. Before you know it all of your clothes have become the new baggy look. Eventually they shrink and now it is the tight look again! It really wasn't me- just played off as "they don't make clothes like they used to!"

GOING DOWNHILL

I didn't ever set out to become obese, I doubt that anyone does. I don't believe that anyone likes being overweight. Being overweight is either something that you have been for your entire life and know no other way, or like me, it snuck up on you. I got in a rut, and eating filled a void in my life. I worked full time, I had a baby to care for, bills that didn't seem to have relief in sight, and a marriage that didn't provide any companionship or romance. I knew no reasons to want to be thin, my husband was more concerned with going out with his friends and being with them. He was never around for that or much of anything else. I was a single mother with two incomes, and a married woman with no husband.

After two years of this lifestyle— and I'd been on a "diet" the entire time— I still had

Some crazy ideas!!

not only not lost any weight, but I was bigger. Desperate and frustrated, I concocted yet another of my "great" ideas. I tried to recruit my very thin friend, Mary, to wear a bikini and carry a sign that said, "AFTER." I, too, would be in a bikini, but with a "BEFORE" sign. Together, we would stand on a busy street corner soliciting drivers for donations for my LIPOSUCTION FUND! I really thought that it would work! (What's with me and bikinis and signs?)

How is it with all these great ideas and energy, weight loss never worked for me before now? A woman I met at a pool party mentioned that she owned an aerobics studio and that she thought I was too pretty to carry around all that extra weight. She offered help if I wanted her to. Help me what? Get a partner to share my life with? Help me be more understanding of my husband and his lifestyle? What?! Was she implying that I was fat? She must be blind! I had my new gold trimmed swim suit on, with a towel draped ever so carefully as to camouflage my thighs. No one could see that I was fat— "I was Jane Mansfield-like, Marilyn Monroe-ish , but not overweight!" I thought about what she said, and after my initial rage at her wore off, I decided to exercise at her aerobics studio. I attended classes three to four times a week, dying each time I noticed one of the hunk bodybuilder guys in the gym checking out the women in class— the skinny women in spandex. I prayed they wouldn't notice me (how could they not!), at least not until I lost some weight!

She gave me a print out of a diet she recommended— the typical 3 meals a day, snacks thrown in, lots of veggies, fruit and a lot of brown rice! The usual seven- day-a-week plan, every meal for you to follow. "Too rigid and too much food for me," I thought. I looked at that "diet" and thought it would make me gain weight! It called for more food in a meal than I ate all day! Sure, it didn't call for ice cream, but even *I* thought it was too much food, with too strict a regimen! What did these experts know anyway! I obviously wasn't ready.

Trying every plan

I knew what I needed to do! "Begin eating only a bran muffin"— (which is secretly packed with 25 or more grams of fat!), for breakfast, and a salad the rest of the day! That didn't last long. Soon I had stopped exercising (I was convinced the laughter from the gym had to be the hard bodied guys laughing at the obese woman dancing around and jiggling as she went!) and I was overeating again. More excuses to avoid the changes I didn't want to face. Besides, I had a good excuse— there were too many meals in her plan.

Eventually, after numerous diets with no results, I had resigned myself to "fatdom." Jenny® didn't work for me. I spent weeks of my time and hundreds of dollars buying all of the prepackaged food, eating it as directed. I thought that it tasted ok. I made myself eat it- and a little extra here and there (her food is low cal so a bit more couldn't hurt, right?!). I went to the behavior modification classes— I cheated, I quit. It wasn't for me. "Nutri-" was next. Their food left me 10 pounds heavier, and hundreds of dollars poorer. I think I believed that if I spent money, a lot of money, on a particular system that I would feel obligated to stick with it. I didn't want to waste money. Mine or dad's, as he often encouraged me to diet by sending me to these places as well.

"Julia, you just failed at every diet you ever tried, what are you going to do?".... ***I'm going to Disney World!*™"**

I took Taylor to Disney® for some fun and a break from reality.. After getting back and seeing the few photos we had taken, I went back to feeling depressed, and trying more diets. ***Looking back, I'm sure I could have been one of the characters—I was as big as this one!!***

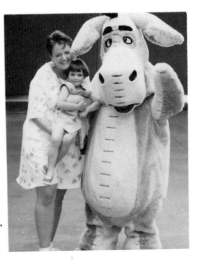

I really wanted any of them to work. Like being in college, I considered myself a student— even if I wasn't learning, I must be getting smarter being there! The problem was that they offered their variety of sweets. "Nutri-" had little sweet tart like treats, very few of them, so I would supplement with a few real sweet tarts—

what could it hurt? Every diet book that I bought offered little help. I would stock my house with bags of groceries, only to have them spoil before I would get to them. I brought a blender to work and tried the Opti- something liquid diet. **I really just wasn't ready to take charge of my life, attempting to surrender myself to these plans.**

One of my role models, Oprah, did it, and she wheeled a wagon load of fat across her stage. She was wearing jeans again. I would do exactly what she did. I was successful, I achieved my objective. I lost a lot of weight, and then I gained all of my weight back and some. I did just what Oprah did!

My office mate at the time made unmerciful fun of me to everyone and lied when he told our boss that I turned my blender on when he was on the phone with a client. He was perhaps the meanest of all about my weight. I thought he supported my diet, but behind my back he ridiculed me to all who would listen to him. "Julia on another of her ridiculous diets that she won't stick with!" he would say. I lost all credibility with everyone who knew me, they were sick of hearing about me go on and on about my desire to be thin, while watching me eat a pastry or gorge on whatever food someone had brought in the office to share. **While the desire was there, I expected someone else to do it for me!**

Even though I thought my face was still pretty, I refused to try on clothes at stores for fear I'd see my rear end in one of those three-way mirrors—a sight that would depress me for days. I ordered my clothes from mail order catalogs. If no one saw me buy a size 22 pair of pants or the XX shirts, they wouldn't know I wore that size, right?! I really believed that as long as my clothes were dresses and baggy that people wouldn't really notice how big I was getting. For parties and holidays I always bought a new outfit and accessories, I thought it was great camouflage! Dress me up and hide behind my clothes. It must have worked to some degree, there are those who say to me now that I 'never seemed that big,' although they're probably just being nice. What a relief. It must have been that the movie theater seats were made too small, not me getting too big!

I really thought that I was trying to eat right. I was beginning to believe it must be my metabolism that was the culprit, not my fault! I would watch the way a large woman* (*definition— anyone bigger than I was!) at my office would have a bag of cookies, sweets, chips, M&Ms® and more, open on her desk and grazing from them all day long! I wasn't doing this, so I must be eating right!

I would have *Lite* ice cream, good fresh bread with real butter, salad bar lunches, bakery goods—not the packaged junk food! Why wasn't I losing weight? I figured that she and I could help each other. I used to occasionally ask her if she wanted to go on a diet with me, for buddy system support. She never took me up on my offer. It wasn't until a few years later I found out that she hated me for doing that. She couldn't believe that I actually thought she needed to diet and then dared to mention it to her. She was happy with her body. I assumed if I was roughly 50 lbs. less her size and miserable about my weight, then she must be totally depressed! My intentions were good, but I hurt her. She was happy with her body and her life. I couldn't see why she wouldn't want to be smaller and healthier, heck it consumed my thoughts! I have to realize that she is happy the way she is. She used to drive a small sports car, so I thought that was a sign of sorts that she deep down wanted to be smaller as well. I learned a lesson though, that setting an example works better than offering someone help. What you see may not be what they see:

I learned my lesson. A person has to want to change, I can't make anyone change! I hope that you can relate to my story, and take something from it that will help you with your change. Spare yourself any agony, like what I went through! You will see how easy managing what you eat can be! I am living proof that what I did works, I have lost 130+ pounds and have kept if off for over 4 years at this writing! I must be onto something that the "experts" haven't figured out yet! **You must look inside for your motivation and drive to succeed before you embark on any change. It has been said that your "why" for doing something is almost everything, making your "how" to do that something as plain as your hand in your face!**

My former boss (not at the airline) once offered me $10 for every pound I lost. Sounds generous, but it made me feel like a high-priced filet that could earn $1000 losing weight. It amazes me how people feel that they can treat you because you are overweight. I know that my boss would never have dreamed of offering an employee who was in a wheelchair $10.00 a step if he could just walk again, yet he didn't think twice about humiliating me with his offer. I was fairly vocal about wanting to lose weight, and always talking about my new diet or fitness plan. Regardless of that, his offer was inappropriate. The money was a big carrot in front of me, and I really thought that this time I would succeed. I would succeed. I had the outfits that I would buy with the money, already picked out of a Victoria's Secret™ catalog! **Again, looking outside before starting within will always leave you short of your goals!**

But, I didn't get the money, because I didn't do it! I was further humiliated in front of my coworkers. In fact, I believe I gained weight in the process! The night he made my the offer, I stopped by my favorite bakery and bought pastries to eat before starting the big "$10/lb. Diet!" (bet that's one you haven't gone on!). What an irony? I was rewarding myself with food, for an accomplishment that I hadn't reached, and one which was not supposed to include food as a reward!

I even stopped for some Lite Ice Cream and once home, my then husband dared to ask for some—I became furious. Why did he need to eat my lite ice cream, he wasn't dieting?" I really thought I could stuff myself, do some aerobics and lose weight! In the process, I couldn't understand why I wasn't getting thin! What the heck was wrong with me—did thin people obsess about their weight constantly?

My weight wasn't the only thing on a constant roller coaster. My mood, attitude, and work production level all were tied to my weight. I hated the scale because it would dictate my mood. If the scale indicated I had gained a few pounds, my mood and morale were shot for the day— maybe even the week. I had no energy, no motivation and no willpower. I lived to eat and hated myself for it. I was negative and low tone about everyone and everything in my life. It was always the other guys fault, never mine when something went wrong.

Does this sound familiar to you? Do you find your self living the same self-defeating cycle of action? You get yourself totally motivated to lose the weight. Maybe you even go to the extent (and expense!) of getting a gym membership or buying yet another piece of exercise equipment. Maybe a new book by an expert caught your eye, 'the protein this' or 'buster that'.... You went to the grocery store, loaded up on all of the special foods that your new and final diet insisted was the best and only way to eat. This time you are going to do it, right?! The first morning you wake up, you eat the ½ grapefruit, and 2 eggs, you don't combine carbs with proteins, nor fruits with proteins, or whatever it was that the expert assured you was right. Later that day you even managed to say no to the doughnuts at the office. "Ha," look at all those fools eating doughnuts, you'll show them, you will be thinner than all of them soon! At the end of that long and self sacrificing day, while cooking the dinner for your family while your tuna awaits, you nibble on the kids chicken, and just a bite of the mashed potatoes. Just a little won't hurt you, you were so good today, right!? You can't deny yourself everything! One bite becomes several and before long the tuna can wait for tomorrow, or even worse, you eat it too, so as to stay on track with your program! You'll be better tomorrow!... Been there, done that— more times than I care to mention!!

I was sick of dieting. It just didn't work. Feeling as if I no longer had a life to live, I plodded through an existence where, each day, mentally I was "eating" myself up. I would become anxious about meals— every meal, thinking about food more than about any other aspect of my life. It consumed me rather than me consuming it! "Did I each too much? How I can I still be hungry after eating all my lunch? Why did I overeat again— I can hardly move!" Decisions about food made me anxious and if I made a "good" decision (to eat a healthy, low-calorie food or small portion), I was preoccupied with how hungry I was and how unsatisfied it made me feel. If I made a "bad" decision, I felt guilty, hated myself and continually beat myself up about it the rest of the day. If I went on a diet, I constantly thought about food, how much I could eat and when.

The only real joy that I had during these years was coming home to my precious little girl— she didn't care if mama was fat! She loved me for me. She was my approval, my acceptance of who I was. And watching her grow was the best time I had ever known. I loved playing with her and being with her. It just didn't matter if I was fat anymore.

Taking Control of Life!

It's sad how being overweight changes your life, robbing you of interests and activities. Clothes have always been important to me—so much so, that in high school, I was voted runner-up for "Best Dressed" in my senior class. OK, I was voted most talkative, too, are you surprised? Just think, you are only reading my words and you can do that at your own pace. But I love talk to people, especially everywhere I go today!

I never imagined that during my life I would have "fat years," much less hide out in big shirts and leggings, who

Working 9-5

did I think I was fooling? I remember constantly pulling at the back of my shirt to make sure that it was covering my rear end, the part of my body that managed to house most of the 125 pounds of extra Julia!   One day, I wore what I thought a very chic, two piece, oversized purple shirt and leggings. I arrived at work, late as usual, everyone was already around the conference room table. As I made my way to a seat, one of my male co-workers turned to greet me and actually said, "Look, here comes Barney!" They all, even my boss, burst out laughing! I wanted to crawl under the nearest rock. Rather than shrink away, I joined in on the fun. I made some remark about him, and how it was sad that he had to resort to making fun of me in order to divert the attention away! I had them roaring with laughter, verbal sparing, I was becoming a master at it. I never let them see me cry, I wouldn't dare. As the only woman in an all male sales force, not to mention the fact that I out produced all of them, I had to be one of the guys, and join in the fun even if it was at my expense!

I was reminded recently of another story from that office. An older gentleman who worked there, noticed my wedding picture on my desk, and like all brides, I looked great that day. This man saw the picture of the thin, young, beautiful bride and told me that "my daughter made a beautiful bride." My daughter? She was only three and certainly not married yet. No, the bride he was referring to was me, and he didn't know it! He definitely needs glasses and some sensitivity classes as well!

Resigned to being fat ☹

As the years went by, I had all but given up that I would be thin ever again. Oh sure, there was always a new diet or plan that I was determined would work for me, it just never did. Everyone else seemed to be able to eat a Big Mac™, but when I did it was only me that got big, or so I thought! At this point, I was pretty sure that it must be my metabolism or perhaps I was genetically predisposed to being obese.

One fall, I was broke as usual and decided to have a garage sale. I sold old toys, wedding gifts that we had never used, clothes that Taylor had outgrown, all of my old leather skirts and pants and clothes sized 10. Resigned to the fact that I was and always would be fat, I sold my wardrobe of boutique outfits I had collected from shops all over the country during my thin years. My garage sale reaffirmed my love for sales— *A young man just out of college was looking for dishes. I had a set of Chinese food service for four. I assured him that my Chinese dishes were in fact perfect for his needs. "Forget cereal bowls," I told him, "with these you can create a mood!" I described for him the results he could expect when bringing a girl and Chinese take out food back to his place, whipping out his authentic Chinese dishes. "She will be so impressed and will be putty in your hands!" He of course gladly bought the dishes!*

The garage sale went great. I made a few hundred dollars.

Taking Control of Life!

To celebrate, I took Taylor for ice cream and shopping. Of course, adding to my vice of eating was shopping! All things that I look back on as actions that were meant to make me 'feel good.' I typified the phrase..... nothing exceeds like excess. I was going to just settle with being this way. Of course, I wasn't thinking ahead more than a day with my life.

Now that my stylish thin wardrobe was gone, I thought I had better accept the fact that I would look like a "matronly housewife" for the rest of my life. Feeling the need to spice up my outlook on life as well as my marriage, I went to Glamour Shots® to have pictures taken for my then-husband. I really looked forward to the photo session and giving a picture of myself to him. I remember thinking I was still pretty. After all, my husband often told me that I was the prettiest fat lady he knew! (That proves that he loved me, right?). I felt attractive as I sat through the makeup and hair, then the shoot itself. This was exactly the kind of boost I needed. I thought how easy Cindy Crawford's job must be! I couldn't wait to see the elegant me! The old me! Anticipation quickly turned to disbelief!

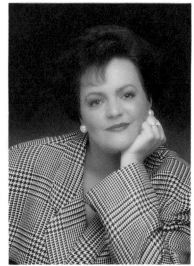

Who was this woman looking back at me from this glossy 5x7? I never showed him the pictures, despite their best efforts. I didn't feel as though I looked good— I looked like a heavy middle aged woman! This wasn't me, it couldn't be- I hadn't gotten that far gone? *I think I weighed 250+ pounds in this photo, at 29!*

I had tried dieting, and each diet ended with me either a little poorer or a little heavier— often both. I was done with all of that. No more disappointments for me!

Stop and think about yourself for a moment. Do any of these stories sound familiar to you? How do you see your body right now, today? How do you picture yourself? Is the picture of yourself realistic? Are you living like I did, convinced that you are trying your best to lose weight while eating the hamburger and fries!? You have to eat, right!? When I was overweight, I always thought, "I'm pretty, and my body doesn't look that bad." For immediate reaffirmation, I'd look around and find someone heavier than me. It's difficult for me to believe (and admit to) that I used to have my young daughter compare me to other overweight ladies. I'd ask her if she thought mommy was slimmer than that lady. We had this nonverbal communication thing going— I would sort of nod in a woman's direction, Taylor would look her up and down, then give me her nod. I was starting to get the "no" nod more than the "yes." "I should get this kid's eyes checked, her vision is getting bad," I thought. At 250 pounds, I wanted to feel "skinny" by some standard, even if my subject for comparison was a 300-pound woman! It made me feel better at the time, but must have been a confusing self-confidence lesson for my little girl! **Don't let your comparison be on the outside— rather look inside to what you are capable of doing, becoming, and achieving!**

Well, a few years later and another 25 pounds heavier, which is only about 6 pounds per year, I was shoe shopping with Taylor and a salesperson asked me "when are you due?" Rather than be a wall flower, I demanded to speak with her manager, and I inquired about training classes in sensitivity for his employees and suggested that this person be sent to one! How dare this sweet little woman ask me such a rude question— I was not 8 months pregnant! I was full figured, large, plus sized, if you will, but not pregnant! I demanded 25% off on my shoes! I seemed to always make my problem the fault of someone else.

A couple of weeks later I was relieved to find out that yes, I was in

Another green light for food!

fact, expecting! I immediately began telling anyone who would listen "I'M PREGNANT!" The translation for this of course, was 'I'm not really fat I'm pregnant!' I believed that pregnancy would somehow excuse my obesity, or that people would think my fat was all baby— even though I was only 8 weeks pregnant! Maybe that sweet little well-meaning saleslady was psychic and knew something I didn't! Well, back to doing what I did best— eating for two!

The pregnancy went well, I didn't gain too much weight this time, *only* 40 or so pounds. I remember my husband saying to me that if I ended up weighing more than him, he would leave me! It was a joke, I didn't take him seriously. (I think I was way passed him already!) Why should I take him seriously? We had been married 6 years now and it was stable. We had a child and one on the way!

Our lives continued to move along as it had in the past, we obviously even managed to have sex once in the past few months. By this point in our marriage, he was hardly ever around. At this point that was ok with me, as Taylor and I had so much fun together. He didn't know what he was missing! Besides, I had all I needed— a loving child who approved of me, and another on the way that I needed to feed to ensure his growth! *What a small universe I was living in.*

During my pregnancy, one winter day, he insisted on going deer hunting for what must have been the 15th time that month. I put my foot down that Friday night (or Saturday morning, as it was 3:00 am when he made it home!) and said— "No, tomorrow you are going to see Taylor sit on Santa's lap with me whether you like it or not! I promised her you'd be there!" He refused and called me a few choice names before falling asleep on the couch.

Frostbite...

I felt particularly feisty that night, as I was upset. After finishing my midnight snack, I got the red food coloring out, and put some on a cotton ball. I proceeded to paint his nose red— brighter than Rudolph's on a cloudy night! I kept thinking that in the morning, he would see it in the mirror and know I meant business, then go back to bed and later accompany his daughter to see Santa. I went to bed, only to awaken and find him gone, no note to telling me he was gone or anything. Hmm... I went about my day. It was a bitterly cold morning, and an hour or so later, in comes the deer hunter, panic stricken and actually frightened! He was exclaiming that he was frostbitten, and his nose had gotten frozen while up in his tree stand. He said he had gone back to his truck to warm up when he noticed his very red nose. Then he raced home so that I could take him to the emergency room. It was *really* red— he feared that he might lose his nose! I fell on the floor, I was laughing so hard I 'nearly soiled myself!' He stood there gazing blankly like one of his beloved deer, eyes caught in the headlights of an oncoming car! I held up my fingers, which were also stained red. Slowly it dawned on him that I was mother winter who had caused his "frostbite." It is sad to say, that was one of the few times we laughed together, although he didn't go to see Santa. It remains one of our better moments together.

THAT MAKES TWO!

Clark Leonard came into the world in August, via a scheduled C-section. Thank goodness, at 270+ pounds I thought labor may have killed me. My best friend Dana drove me to the hospital, my parents bringing Taylor along later. The new father made it in time, and stayed around long enough to take a picture or two. He had to leave soon after I was taken to my room, as he had an important dinner meeting at a nice restaurant in town. Hmm... He was a carpenter, and he only had union meetings to attend? My father couldn't understand what meeting he would have that was more important than getting to know his new baby son! I didn't mind, I had a son to get acquainted with.

He was my little "frog baby"— he resembled a frog when he was born. *(There were many people that made that comment and it stuck with me, or him, at the time.)* Taylor came into this world gorgeous— nurses from other units actually stopped by to see "the precious baby girl." Clark on the other hand was all boy, he didn't want to be mistaken for a girl even for a second. He succeeded. He was so long and skinny that his uncle nicknamed him "Spindles" and made jockey jokes. He was adorable, he was a life to be loved, and I had now another life to focus on without having to think of my own. With two children, my habits were less important, and I could be a child too— with less responsibilities, and all fun! Of course, changing a diaper and feeding— but those are fun, too. Taking focus off me was a relief....again!

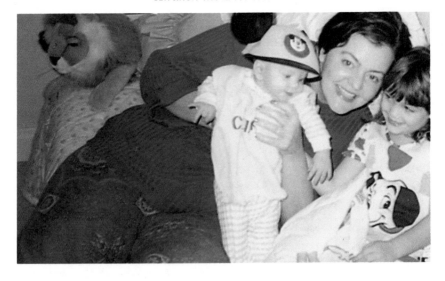

My little 'frog baby' Clark, was my second, born about 4 years after Taylor. This was one of a very few pictures that I manage to find in my album.

Birds of feather

The proud father did come visit each night we were in the hospital, bringing along his ritual evening six pack and of course a friend whose habits were the same. (*Birds of a feather flock together!*) They stayed till the beer was gone and then were on their way. I was upset that he brought beer into the hospital. I vowed that I would die before I would let him turn my son into a beer drinker.

By this point in our marriage, I didn't know which I disliked more— the way being with him made me feel, or the way I felt about myself. He did manage to squeeze in enough time to bring us home from the hospital. He pulled up to the curb in his huge pickup truck, and I had to strain to climb into it. He must have forgotten that I had just had a C-section. In any case we were on our way home.

Once home, I found his best friend (married) lying on the couch in our living room with his new girlfriend. They were making out in front of

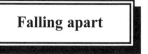

Falling apart

Taylor— 38 years old and acting like teenagers in front of a child! I had a tough time explaining to Taylor why he was kissing a woman that wasn't his wife. They were separated, but none the less Taylor knew them both and was confused. I suspect that he had been seeing her for a while but I wasn't one of my husband's confidants and wasn't informed of the budding romance.

Those two men were I think were up to no good most of the time, but if he had been cheating, I thought my husband would stop it. "We are Catholic, you just don't do that," I thought to myself. My husband then suggested I make a snack for everyone. They were hungry. "Hello? I just came home from having a C-section and have a new baby to take care of!?" I threw a bottle across the room, packed up the diaper bag and against doctor's orders, drove myself to my friend Dana's. *I now realize how true the saying is "show me your friends, and I'll show you— you!"*

The girls and their husbands, and all the kids were there for dinner— much better company and much better care given to the needs of me and the baby!! (They all marveled at how cute "frog-baby" was! I have the sweetest friends. They told me little white lies to make me feel happy!) They were enraged by my husband's lack of sensitivity. All voiced the opinion that I should divorce him. This wasn't the first time I had heard that. I was in no shape mentally or financially to do that! I tuned them out, I didn't want to listen no matter how right they were! What did they know?! They had perfect lives— husbands that not only loved them, but were actually helpful with raising the children, that were good providers and didn't spend more time out with friends than at work. I didn't like my life but I sure didn't want to make it worse. I believed I wasn't worth changing, and saving a marriage would be easier, although at the time not realizing I needed one to have the other.

No job, two kids...
time to remodel?

My carpenter husband was laid off, again, from his job. He decided this would be the ideal time to remodel our house. No money, a new baby and a terrible marriage. I can think of no better time to rip your house apart! Walls were torn out and the stairway to nowhere was built. Weeks went by with very little progress, but lots of mess for me to clean up each night when I returned home from work. When I would get home, it was time for him to leave. He would go to the lumber store in town and then out for a beer. Alone again, but with lots of laundry and cleaning to do, I wouldn't have time to miss him, with diapers and drywall dust to tend to. One day he said a friend had told him a local company was hiring and wondered if we knew anyone worked there. I said my dad knew the CEO fairly well. He said that he had lusted after that job for years but never knew all that I had to do was ask my dad to make a phone call.

I didn't know that he would want to have a job with that company, and he never mentioned it to me. I asked about trying to help him get into a management position in the previous job my dad had gotten him and he got angry with me. He said he was happy being a carpenter, and he implied that I was embarrassed by what he did for a living. I didn't try to help him after that. Now, I mention that dad could make a call for him and he is excited! He said that he had always wanted a job with that company because of how "cush" it was, and how great are the benefits. *He used to joke that the only reason he had married me is he thought my dad would be able to get him a good job.   They say there is a little truth in every joke!*

Well at least things were looking up. With one phone call, dad secured him an interview

On the right track?...

and the job was his for the taking. We would have money, and we could get the addition completed. His stress would lessen and we would be a family! It was high time, with two kids, it would be nice to have someone to share the load with! And somewhere in there, I might even lose a pound or two.

Clark soon started crawling and I worried he would get hurt with all the nails and boards strewn about. "It will be great to have this mess cleaned up and done for good," I thought. The new job's hours were crazy, as he would leave for work at 4:00 am and not get home till 10 or 11 pm. We never saw him. My days were filled with playing with the kids, and eating, and shopping, and eating.

I never did weigh myself after having Clark, the best I can tell you is I know I weighed 265 lbs prior to delivery, but I know that I gained over the next few months after the delivery. I just wasn't caring any longer. My kid's didn't care that mommy was very heavy. They loved me just the way I was. I used to make up bed time stories to tell the kids about their dad, portraying him as a little-boy cowboy. I did it to give the kids memories that included their dad, to make him bigger than life to them.

The videos I took during this era are all kids, no grown ups in them at all.   I was the camera man, and Taylor carried Clark around. We had a lot of fun, but I felt something, or in our case, someone, was always missing.   He was out earning a living, working very hard physically. I was irritable, every time he came home we would have a fight about him never being home. It seemed so illogical even then, we fought about his absence, yet whenever he *was* around it was so unpleasant. So why did I want him home in the first place? Besides, when he was around, I didn't feel like I could curl up on the couch with a half gallon of ice cream, or he would make fun of me. I enjoyed it most when I was alone— me, my sitcoms and my ice cream. I was fine! *(Or so I thought.)*

The few times I'd see myself in a photo, I couldn't believe or accept that it was me. I didn't look like that, did I?! Although I adamantly refused to allow anyone to take my picture, I accepted a friend's gracious offer to take pictures at my son's first birthday party— how very sweet of her! The outfit I wore that day was so cute. I bought a shorts romper from a catalogue and had spent days sewing sequins and pearls. It was so pretty that I knew it would look precious. I served a delicious menu with a fabulous cake, and all my friends and family were there. My spouse was even was there— the perfect family!

"Everyone must be thinking how happy we are— two kids, nice house, new job." The boys all left for about an hour, leaving my dad to play host and work the grill. Thank God for my dad, always there playing the role of co-host with me! They returned and rejoined the party. He gave Clark a fire truck he bought while they were gone. "How sweet, he left to go get his son a gift! He might not be the best host, but he loves the kids." It wasn't until months later I found out the little red fire truck was from "HER!" *(How dare he bring a gift from her to him, to our home!)*

A few days after the party, my friend gave me prints of the pictures she had taken. The back-stabber, the traitor! She revealed the truth...she was no friend, her pictures made me look absolutely huge! The woman in those pictures couldn't be me! I was the picture perfect hostess that day, I had the cutest outfit, the party was a great success. Who was this obese woman in these pictures cutting my son's cake? Not me! I was depressed, I needed more to eat.

The realization slapped me in the face— my gosh, it's ME! I was ashamed to think that the cheerleader and stewardess I used to be had become a matronly, very heavy woman. I wasn't even 30 years old! Of course, you can guess what I did. I ate the rest of the birthday cake that I had hidden in a plastic container in the freezer and pledged to start on a diet... **tomorrow!!**

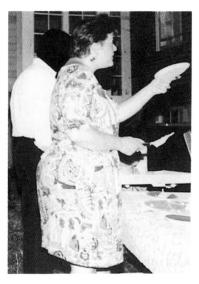

(face covered to protect the guilty, I mean innocent!)

LIFE-CHANGING EVENTS

It wasn't until I took a good, long look at myself that I realized and accepted that I was the lady with the large rear-end and ill-fitting pants. Makeup wouldn't cover up, and new outfits couldn't hide, my obesity. Looking back, it's evident that I hated the way I looked. I have very few— maybe a handful— of pictures of myself holding either of my two precious children. As a matter of fact, very few pictures of me exist at all from my "fat" years. I was in hibernation!

You already know the demise of my marriage and how that facilitated my decision to change. A few other events also contributed to my wanting to finally lose the weight— this time. Some were more subtle than others, this one was downright scary!

"I'm dying!" One afternoon I was at my parents after "the letter" came, trying to figure out how to pick up the pieces of my shattered life. My father was indulging me with one of his wonderful neck massages. He abruptly stopped, announcing that he had felt a lump at the base of my neck! *Not* that he and I are two hypochondriacs, but cancer *was* our immediate diagnosis. While he planned the funeral, I called my doctor for an appointment. I arrived a few days later, and waited nervously in my Dr.'s exam room, picturing the piano-box casket with me stuffed inside, I worried for my children. "Who would raise them? Would they remember me when they were older? Would this other woman raise my little girl, thinking this woman was her mother!? Clark is so little, he won't even remember me!" As I lie there on the table draped in the latest paper gown, I was actually scared. I didn't think of myself as a very strong person, able to handle this like the

Taking Control of Life!

people you read of who battle cancer with such strength and character. I was shallow and self absorbed, and I only had my loyal friends from high school. No one else even wants to be around me, not even my husband. I would die a miserable, lonely, cowardly death. The doctor examined me and arrived rather quickly at a diagnosis, it was.............a FAT DEPOSIT!

Now I actually wanted to die! Cancer would have sounded better! I couldn't even get dying right! I was a mess! A joke! "Everyone makes fun of me and everyone has been laughing behind my back for over 2 years now." More thoughts ran through my head: "My husband's friends have been guests in our home for dinner so many times these past 2 years, all of them knew of the affair and no one stood up for me! Not one of those men chided him when he ridiculed me or called me a nag in front of them for asking where they were off to, all of them knowing he was actually off to spend time with "her." No one made him stop what he was doing to come home to me or to his children. No one is looking out for me!" Least of all me.

I abused myself more than anyone else had. Here I lie, thinking that I had cancer, only to find out the "illness" was of my own making. I actually starting to think that the fault for the problems in my life might actually be of my own making. A thought that I just couldn't handle. I needed a diversion. Not to worry, on the way home I swung by my favorite pastry shop: it's amazing how much my thoughts cleared after a napoleon or two!

Even then I didn't change. I wanted to, and I even thought that I was changing— I was eating less, only sweets rather than a meal with sweets. I knew how pathetic my life was as I was spiraling out of control. It was pretty pathetic.

Awakened by a homeless man!

One night, after getting the kids to bed, having done all of my housework and arguing with my spouse, I went for a drive. I had to get out of there, but I really had no destination in mind, I just drove. I couldn't stand to be in the same house as him after what he did, and was continuing to do! I went to my favorite park, where there are beautiful old Victorian mansions, huge homes filled with happy families— reminders of the 1901 World's Fair. It is a tranquil place. I lived there when I was single when I thought I had the world by the tail. I began thinking, "what happened to me to make me end up this way? I used to have so much fun and really enjoy life. I had so much energy, I used to ride my bike all over the park, just for fun?!" I longed for my old way of life, I longed for the old me.

On the way home I stopped at a gas station for a candy bar, I had a thing for Mounds™ bars. That is where I encountered a man I will never forget. I paid for the candy bar at the little window, the ones that the cashier slides open, keeping you outside, avoiding thieves. I noticed this man sitting by the building, a brown bag in his dirty city-stained hands. He looked up at me and smiled. I felt guilty buying candy when the poor man probably didn't even have dinner, or maybe even a shower. I sheepishly looked away. He wasn't about to let me off that easy! I made my way to my car, pulling my sweatshirt down past my rear-end as I retreated. He shouted to me ***"Girl, you got too much food in you!... That's right, too much food in you!"*** This man with nothing to his name, was telling me my business! How dare he! I got in my car, gesturing to him off as I drove away. To think I was actually feeling sorry for him until he opened his mouth! "Old fool,

Taking Control of Life!

bum," I thought. I soothed the sting of his humiliation with the delicious coconut filling. But as soon as I had driven far enough away that I was sure no one who had heard him would be able to see me, I cried. I cried and thought of what he had said. I thought about my life, and I cried for what seemed like hours.

It was during this moment that, looking back I know I was hitting bottom. My life had to change because I felt it couldn't get worse. And even if it could, I knew I couldn't feel any worse about myself. I can only imagine how someone whose addictions are more severe would feel hitting bottom— an alcoholic for instance. The pain, though, was enough for me that I didn't want anymore.

I think about that man often. He was right! He didn't lie, he didn't slander me, he didn't say it to hurt my feelings, he was merely calling it as he saw it. This man was just observant of the world around him, and probably has to be. I imagine his survival depends on his skill of observation. He was right. He didn't my gesture to him! He pointed out what was wrong with me— I had too much food in me, plain and simple! He didn't say that I was an axe murderer, a thief, or child abuser. He merely said that I had too much food in me! He didn't know that I had a marriage that wasn't working, or problems with acceptance. All he could tell was what he could see with his own eyes. I was self destructing, stuffing myself way beyond capacity. I had too much food in me! I knew that it was my own decisions, and my own happiness that only *I* can be responsible for, not anyone else!

It is a pretty simple concept if you think about it. You can pour water into a glass; it fills up, and if you don't stop, it will overflow. The human body, unfortunately, isn't as efficient at getting rid of extra food as the glass is at letting out excess water. Our bodies store it up; in big, ugly, chunky globs tucked under our skin— orange peel like in appearance that it is not pleasant! The old master painters had a gift for making obese women look like beautiful cherubs. That is great for artwork, but in a bathing suit, in today's society, it just doesn't look as beautiful!

PART

II

Taking Control of Life!

SELF-ANALYSIS

*The first step in taking control of life is looking at yourself— ask yourself if you "have too much food in you." It is starting with a look there first, then within you for the guidance and strength necessary for change. Because once fat is there, it wants to stay! You have to eat less and exercise in order to loose fat from your body. It doesn't end there: you have to eat right and exercise **forever** to **keep** it off. That is the truth, there is no other way to do it! As my sister told me many times, "a moment on the lips, a lifetime on the hips!" Are you willing to begin making a commitment that will be a difficult challenge, yet will reap tremendous rewards? Only you can find the answer to this question within you.* And find it you must!

An American disease?

Many estimates report obesity as a disease— ranked the 2nd leading cause of preventable death in our country. How can something be a disease, yet be preventable? If you can prevent something, yet you still do it, it is then self-inflicted! Don't stuff your body with too much food and you won't be obese. I wish cancer was that easy to cure! Rather, as a society, we spend billions of dollars a year on weight loss products and programs, yet we continue getting fatter!

It is estimated that 75% of us are on a diet at any given time, trying to cure our self-made disease! Wouldn't it be a better world if we all put our energy and perspectives in the right place and simply quit putting too much food in our bodies? The dieting seventy-five% of us could then join the other 25% who are spending their lives doing more important things than dieting. Perhaps they are trying to find cures for real diseases, or

Taking Control of Life!

volunteering their time helping make our world a better place. **Did you know in a laboratory study, rats that ate less food on a daily basis lived much longer than those that were allowed to eat unlimited quantities?** — we're not rats, I know I want to live longer!

It's a lifestyle, not a diet!

Dieting is a waste of time and energy! Put your efforts into something really important and watch and see how much time goes by before you realize you have been so busy you actually forgot to eat! That is a great feeling— **that is the key to successful weight loss! Food has to become less important than you and the contributions you make in your own life and the world around you!** You have God-given talents and contributions to make in this world- don't let them go untapped! Live the life, not the diet!!

One of the great realizations I had is that I was eating a lot of unhealthy, fattening foods. Once I cut some of it out, added more healthy foods, the weight started peeling off, with little effort or work. Best of all, no crazy diets to follow! If you weigh 250 pounds or more, you are probably eating a lot of food—a lot! *Cut back on the portions, eliminate some of the fat and you will amaze yourself at how easily the weight comes off!*

How many times have you said to yourself, "I'll eat whatever I want today and start my diet tomorrow"? You know the result: you binge all day, starve yourself the next, eat moderately on day two, and by day three you can no longer resist having a candy bar or other "forbidden" food. After eating the forbidden food you think, "Well, I blew my diet now, so I might as well eat anything I want!" So, you eat everything in sight! Disgusted with yourself, you vow to "go back on your diet tomorrow." But tomorrow never comes! I know that this is true for many more people than just me! Believe me, I have studied this phenomenon! Ok, not scientifically, but as a street scientist!

Recently I gave a copy of my first book and some supplements I use, to an acquaintance of mine. I saw him a few days later and asked how it was going. He told me 'I'm going on my diet tomorrow.' Because he cheated at breakfast that morning, his thinking was 'the day was shot!' so I have failed today. You know there is not a clock, or a position of the sun that needs to determine when we start making healthy decisions. Again, I am not talking about a diet, I am referring to *a lifestyle*. The supplements I gave him are an easy thing to take— but inside he wasn't ready to make the commitment. Perhaps I didn't make that point strongly enough in the first edition, so let me say it again, **do not go on another diet, not ever again!**

It's your choice!

So what if my acquaintance made a "bad" decision as to what food he should eat for breakfast. Why should that force him to gorge for the rest of the day, until the magical tomorrow approaches and he can again attempt "dieting." He is still a nice person, he didn't decide to rob the bank he works at, he merely ate a doughnut! The day was young, he had the rest of the day to make healthier decisions rather than continue to eat fattening foods until the magical 'diet hour' approached and it was the mystical "tomorrow!" I can tell you that even now if I feel I ate an extra something, I will just make a point to spend an extra 5 minutes on the stationary bike or doing aerobics. Of course, it's much easier to just make the right decisions. (*Maintaining requires making the right choices on a daily basis, too!*)

Of course, **deciding** that you will start making healthy

decisions now is the first and best step to living life well! Doesn't this approach seem slightly more logical than *announcing* the start of a diet!? "Attention shoppers, I am on a diet; yes that's right starting this morning in aisle 3, I am now on a diet!" That is just silly! It doesn't matter what you ate 10 minutes ago, 3 hours ago or 3 years ago (because you can't change it). The only thing that matters is what you eat next or don't! Why does sleep need to separate the end of something and the beginning of the next. It doesn't! It's all in your mind. **Living with a strong sense of purpose in life comes from within, and will give you the strength to make the right choices!**

You can't change or control what is in the past, you're only able to control what you decide to do in the present and future! Right now, today is the first day of the rest of your life. How do you want to live it, what kind of body do you want to live it in? You don't necessarily need to look at your next action being one which you eat healthy. It could be to take a walk, ride a bike, or focus on something or someone else that will take the focus off of food. Any action that you take, be it writing down your goal for the week, will be a positive move.

How do you stop this vicious cycle? I know that for me the change was brought about by a collection of humiliating experiences. I don't have all the answers, but I do know this—if TODAY you start caring about yourself more than you do about food; caring about your health, realizing that you are in control of what goes into your mouth; begin taking pride in your appearance, and living with a meaningful purpose in life, then each day will get easier to make those right choices about not only what you eat, but in all that you do. You've got to picture the person inside that you know can accomplish great things in life. By calling on the energy deep inside to break the barriers holding you back from doing anything you want, you will move mountains!

You're in control!

When you realize that you are in control here, you will realize that change is within your grasp! Before you know it, people will notice a change in you and your demeanor. They'll compliment you, and soon you won't need it because you'll be complimenting yourself. You will begin to like the person you are!! No one can make you feel as good about yourself as you can. Before long, you'll not only feel good about yourself, but you'll look great, too!

Realize that you have too much food in you, and cease stuffing yourself—it is in your power! It's amazing how a picture changes when only we change on the inside—our thoughts and perspectives. Pretty soon, everyone begins to see the picture we started to see long ago. If I ever find that homeless man, I owe him a huge debt of gratitude, and an apology!

Let's start today. What should you do right now to get going? .... You've been reading for all of 30 minutes, this book must not work!.....Julia doesn't know what the heck she is talking about! You want to get a refund right?! No, you're not thin yet—but guess what? You just spent 30 minutes focusing on YOU and not food, and that's a great start! Maybe my rambling thoughts have even made you think a little about your situation or fearful of what may come if you don't change— like the ghost of Christmas yet to come! I hope so. Ultimately all of this is up to you, and you alone. I can be your coach, but you are the only one able to stop yourself from eating that next cheeseburger or pastry, and picking yourself up and becoming more active!

There is a point I want you to remember each day. Because each moment prior to this one is a moment lived— it becomes a

Taking Control of Life!

memory. And therefore each day becomes one, too. But this moment, now, here today is one which you can make the decision to think good thoughts, choose healthy food, and tap into your God-given abilities and talents. Remind yourself each day that...

**"Today is the first day
of the rest of my life!"**

Don't let another day or moment go by without taking one small step to improving who you are. Just by making one small choice that is good, healthy, and positive, in 2 weeks you see noticeably magnificent changes. Don't believe me?

Let me ask you this....Do you imagine that there are things that you would do, or ways in which your life would be different if only you were thinner? If the answer is yes, you are not alone! We all imagine that the grass is greener on the other side! The beauty of this analogy put to weight loss, is that you can do those things right now! You don't have to wait until you are thin to go to the park, to go swimming, to take an exercise class—you can do it now......and it they will only help you in reaching your goal sooner! If we were talking about imagining yourself rich, well that takes time and a lot of work to accomplish. You are lucky! The things that you want out of life as a thinner person are easily attained—and actually doing those things gets you thin! Then the little black dresses and tight (purposely!) jeans will follow!

In this instance.....Visualization meeting Action =Results!!

Making the Change

Sometimes, usually when we least expect it, life changes course. The goings may be rough—especially in the beginning. Once we take command of the new circumstances, we can manage to move ahead and create something good amidst the chaos. The day my life changed, I received an anonymous letter with a brief but devastating message informing me that my marriage was most likely over. In an instant, I had lost what I perceived to be the only remaining socially accepted measure for my self-image. I was no longer someone's wife. I really believed that those looking at my life wouldn't judge me harshly because I was married, felt apart of society, therefore not "dis-functional." Not that *I* was different. Of course, all along I was needing other's approval, and forgot about my own. It was time that my own approval came first—establishing a set of healthy principles to live by!

Although there shouldn't be any one aspect of happiness that should be a measure of your own life. There are a many things that can make us happy, but only for a moment—like my ice cream! What will determine happiness, is when you can look back— at one day, one week, one year, maybe even a decade or two—and realize that the choices you have made are those that were the ones that gave your life its greatest fulfillment-as a solid, caring person. That is happiness! It is your life, not those who may, or may not, approve of it!

Now, I was going to be on my own, the challenge really scared me. I didn't like what and who I had become, not just that I was overweight, but I had let myself become selfish and mean—which I clearly see in hindsight. Needless to say it was obvious there was no place to go but up—at least mentally. It took me awhile to just get myself and my thoughts together. My emotions climbed from being extremely low, to being angry. I was stuck on anger for awhile, but it allowed me to harness the energy to get moving forward for the better. I looked within for strength.

If you allow anger to remain, it eats you up inside, and can cause even more health problems. I was tired of people feeling sorry for me, and more importantly, I was sick of feeling sorry for me! Sympathy is not a healthy emotion- it is a shallow attempt to foster attention to yourself, and it does no one any good, least of all the recipient.

Eventually I began to rise above the anger into more constructive and healthy emotions. I am glad that I did. Like my dad told me, it was time to get my house in order! He didn't mean the unfinished construction mess-of-a-house that the kids and I were living in, he meant me- spiritually, emotionally, and of great concern to him, physically!

At that point, for the first time in a long time, I didn't want to sit and stuff my face, I didn't want eat! I felt the need to do something, make some

Making unhealthy acts the enemy!

changes, that seemed like a good place to start. Food, the major source of pleasure in my life for the past seven years, provided no solace, only painful memories—and the pain exceeded any pleasure I derived from it before. Something *inside* finally changed. I realized that the pints of low-fat ice cream, on which I use to binge, never were a true, consoling friend. Now they became my worst enemy. From that moment, I made a pledge to myself to change my life—for me. The desire to overcome my situation to live a more meaningful life became a strong motivator.

I hope that my words wake you up, I really don't want you

to have to wait for your rock bottom to come along— it might be tragic like mine. If you haven't figured out by now, my unhappiness with my body manifested itself into every aspect of my life. It consumed me! I was a very negative person. Everything bad was always someone else's fault! I let the pity I felt for my obesity absolve me of all responsibility towards others! I felt like the world owed me, since my life wasn't turning out at all as I had planned! Instead, I look back and everything was the opposite of what my wishes were:

Wanting more out of life!

I wanted to star in a soap opera when I grew up; instead I lived one. I wanted to be rich; instead I made my creditors wealthy! I wanted a good marriage and happy well-adjusted kids, Now we're another divorce statistic! I wanted a body like Demi Moore, I resembled the pre-weight loss Roseanne! Even at 265 lbs., when the girls and I would fantasize about who would play each of us when the blockbuster hit of our life story was made, I actually would claim Demi as my look-a-like! **Make your ambition to want more for yourself!!**

I wanted more out of my life than I had managed to get so far! I took some serious inventory, I realized a lot of the things about myself that I didn't like and I decided to change them for the better, forever! That is the great thing about being human, we are our own screenplay writers. You have the ability at any moment to do a re-write with the rest of the screenplay. Change the character that you are playing, or give the character that you are a new persona or a new body in which to play it. And always striving for something greater than where you are is a great thing— it gives you the passion for life! *(That doesn't mean not being happy along the way with your achievements, only that you are always looking to better each area of your life.)*

THE MOST valuable commodity!

It dawned on me that my body had absolutely nothing to do with me- my spirit, my soul, me if you will. Yet, I let my unhappiness with my body cloud every move I made for years! Identifying that you have a problem is the first step to correcting it. You won't change if you truly don't have enough reasons to! Make the decision today to make the next food you eat a healthy choice, even the next thought you have a positive one, not a self-defeating one! How can right now can be your rock bottom, your turning point? The one thing that is most precious to everyone, that will help change take place now is...**TIME!** I looked back and knew that I had used many years of my life doing things that I wouldn't look back on and be proud of— **realizing that helped motivate me upward!**

Realize that now if you don't change, the misery will only get gradually worse. Realize that YOU are far more important than the food that you eat! If you understand that now, if you admit the pain that a few, or hundreds, of pounds are causing you, the thorn will able to stick you to get you started. In other words, ***don't waste any more time of your life!*** Time is running out, make every day count!!

overeating and make a difference in the world! In any case, don't wait to be on your death bed asking for a second chance. **Take each waking day as another opportunity to do the right thing! You don't ever know how many are left!**

Moving On

By taking the initiative and creating positive change in your life today, you will feel so much better about yourself. Or as someone once said: "Change will do you good!" You will believe in your ability to succeed with each small step that you make toward your goal! Think about how great you feel when you complete a task at hand, or a chore you have been dreading. This is no different! Each day, as you begin to take actions that will get you closer to your goal, that is an accomplishment! Be proud of what you have succeeded in, and relish in it! Reward yourself for it! Stop beating yourself over something that happened in the past - reward yourself with an extra 30 minutes on a treadmill or a walk. Be proud at what you do that *is* right! This can make a big difference in your life! We set up positive reward systems for our children— get an 'A', get a treat; do their chores, get an allowance. You too can be guided by the carrot, and a bit moved by the stick. Pretty soon, it becomes second nature, and pleasure of a successful day, week, or month is great!

If you set up this system of positive rewards for yourself, not only in regard to what you eat, but all areas of your life— you will succeed! We really are programmed to strive for that which makes us feel good. You just have to condition your mind initially to believe that the rewards are more pleasing than the foods that you are used to. Rewards and healthy living honestly are better for you. You will become conditioned to love life and have a passion for it, thereby increasing the quality!

Many people suggest that when starting a weight-loss program you stand naked in front of a full length mirror and take inventory of your body. Why make yourself more depressed than you are already? My advice? Do it! If you are like I was and have convinced yourself that you aren't that heavy. Do you have too much food in you? Have you lost control over the appearance of your body? Don't let this sight upset you too much, very few people, even thin ones, look like the "perfect body" without clothes (only those supermodels!). *You* know how you look. You may be able to hide from it all day, but *you* know. It is time to take an honest inventory and give yourself a state of the union speech! It is important to define where and what you want to improve (and, of course, why!). Then you can take action. If you can learn to adapt to the ***self-improvement through self- motivation*** way of creating a positive self-empowering snowball effect for your life, before you know it you will LOVE looking in mirrors and feel proud of a more slim, smiling figure looking back at you! The better you treat yourself, the more dignity and respect that you demand for yourself, the more that you focus on the quality of life, the better you will naturally treat your body!

Today, when I tell people my weight loss story, often they don't believe me. I usually hear, "You? No way! You never weighed 270 pounds." (As if anyone lies about having been obese!) I am glad I have a few pictures to prove that I was once obese! People often comment that not only am I thinner, I look 10 years younger as well! They are a good reminder for me that gives me an added motivation for staying healthy! I keep my old driver's license in my wallet for a quick reference of my past— for myself as well as those with whom I speak during my travels. I almost don't remember what I felt or looked like at 270 lbs. Distant are the memories of hiding my face as I shopped at the plus size stores, or the lonely nights spent in front of the TV eating another fi gallon of ice cream! It may be hard to remember some things, but I know the pain of that experience and the pleasure from living well, will keep me from ever going back there again.

Not barney, but..?

Life is so rewarding and full now. I love my new life, and you'll love yours! I remember all too well, the feeling of despair when I had resigned myself to forever looking matronly. I may have resigned myself to that, but it never made me happy! At dinner recently a 6 year old girl told her mother that she thought I was "Baby Spice." Me!?......a woman who not long ago weighed 270 pounds, who felt miserable, who people called "Barney?"— I almost screamed "YES!" right there in the restaurant. I thought, well, I guess there's nothing wrong with being sexy and a mother. At 36, I look better than I did at 21— I'll take that any day of the week! I love the fact that I am described by even one person as youthful, intelligent and even sexy! I had convinced myself I was going to be matronly for the rest of my life. This is one instance that I am very glad I was wrong!

There are so many wonderful life experiences you miss when you're overweight, at least I did! Simply because you feel you would look ridiculous or wouldn't fit in, sitting meekly by watching other people live the life that you long for! Why do you think that America has become the nation of television junkies that we have? It's a lot easier to watch someone do something and be excited about it then doing it ourselves. Do you think Mark McGuire would have had the *same* feeling watching Sammy Sosa break the Roger Maris home run record, if he had not himself experienced actually *doing* it?! What's more fun and fulfilling, doing something outstanding or watching others do it? Or making your *own* great accomplishments, and also being able to enjoy others', knowing you've experienced the hurdles involved to make those achievements.

Don't lose your energy and passion for life! Lounging on

the sofa eating chips, cookies, pizza and ice cream watching the "stars" ACT out perfect, wonderful and funny "dream" lives instead of being apart of the real picture, has too many people living outside of reality!! Steven Spielberg is good at creating that fantasy for us. Rather than be active participants in life, we have become a world of spectators!

DON'T *BE A SPECTATOR IN LIFE, BE A DOER!!* *If you follow some basic guidelines, you will have the opportunity to do everything on your wish list. Each day, from now on, you will be using you energy to get back into life. It's time to be an active player, not a spectator watching others have fun.*

Going snow skiing, racing down the slope of a mountain, the wind rushing through your hair, your adrenaline flowing that is one heck of a lot better than the filling of a Twinkie™!! You don't believe me? Try it, and then tell me I was wrong. I promise you, you won't be able to! Now that you know you can't turn back, let's get to what I know will help you on the road in style!

GETTING IN THE PICTURE

I do so many things that just a few short years ago I would have never dreamed of doing! Silly, fun things like going down the slide at the park with my two children, or jumping on a trampoline with them. Remember that I mentioned I had so few pictures of me with my children when they were little? I am so proud of this picture. I actually asked someone to take a picture of me with my children. I felt pretty and fit and when I saw the picture, I was pleased. I really like the way that I look now. I am now a part of and in the pictures taken at holidays and events. Not *only* because I want to be, but because I'm not always the cameraman either! It is a great feeling knowing that I am creating a picture of life that I can look back on and be happy with! As well as knowing that I am setting a good example to live by for my children!

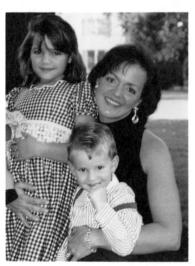

This photo was taken after most of my weight loss, and I was really feeling a sense of peace and happiness with my home and family. I was so happy to be with them having my picture taken. ***Two very special people to me!***

Taking Control of Life!

Another aspect of this argument that I would like to briefly touch on is your family, specifically your children. If you are leading a

A child's health

sedentary life, odds are you are passing that example down to your children. Take a good long look, are your children fat, plump, still hanging on to that 'baby weight' even though they are 10 now?! Is that fair to do to them. And I do mean *to* them!

If you were overweight as a child, take yourself back there for a moment. Try to remember the pain that you felt when the kids teased you. Help your child avoid that pain! It is not too late for them, don't let them waste another day by not learning about healthy eating habits! You are their mentor, their role model. Women tell me: "I can't cook all these healthy meals. I have to feed my family, too?" Are they any less entitled to a long and healthy life than you? You have to lead and teach by example! It is your responsibility to them! I know at one point my children weren't eating the healthy meals they needed. Be mad, be upset, use that anger to stir you into action! Be mad at the chips, the ice cream, the ad companies that make it all seem soooooo good! Don't be mad at yourself, be proud of yourself that you realized it now, before it was too late—and change! That is all that is required of you now, in order that you may ***awaken the diet within you!!***

Your kids are important to you, I'm sure. You want them to look back and see you in their pictures from parties and gatherings. I know because I was embarrassed to be in a picture, there aren't the memories that a photo can create. On the other hand sometimes I am glad they don't see the heavy me back then. Don't let your image or self esteem keep you from being in the picture—the picture of life!

FOOD BASICS 101

Now, here's the secret, here's all that you have to do, Go on a rigid diet, watch every bite you eat. Measure and weigh all your food. Don't combine sugars with proteins, guavas with mangos, no Twinkies® with pizza, no sherbert. Go to an expensive health food store and load up on exotic groceries and $20 bottles of herbs that you can't even pronounce..! Get into a zone, don't use the phone, break through this and breath like that!   **NO!!!!!!!**

Doesn't that sound like every diet book out there? I have one written by a major star, it has the most elegant pictures and recipes that sound too good to be true, but I couldn't figure out exactly what it was she was suggesting that I do. It had phases, groups, dangers of combining this with that. I am not the smartest of people, granted, but I couldn't figure out what she meant! I loved the pictures though and even thought the recipes looked great. However, I don't have hours to spend in the kitchen, and don't believe in spending time that way, so away the book went to my land of misfit diet books— all with too rigid a program or too complicated one! Isn't that why you got this book, so that you could have someone tell you exactly what they think you have to do to organize your life, your eating and your thoughts? I give you a lot more credit than that! My plan for you is a lot more basic and simple than all that!

Realize that you are in control of what you eat, how you make it and under what conditions you choose to eat! Now's the time for taking back control of YOUR life, and get into the picture, too!   Madison Avenue with all of it's ads for big sized meals that you can't live without has had control of what you eat long enough! Goodbye to compulsive eating, hello to controlled eating. You don't need to be told what to eat and what exactly not to eat. It starts with learning to *LIVE!*

If you have been overweight your entire life and were never taught healthy eating habits, you really should go to a nutritionist. Your doctor can refer you to one. Tell them you don't want them to put you on a diet, you just want facts about what is good for your body and what isn't. While you're at it, ask them why the government's food pyramid recommends so many starches. And why they put out a new Body Mass Index that claims we are all obese! They push starches on us, we get fatter. Then they call us fat and tell us it's our fault! Some things are just so obvious, yet we have so many freedoms that many of our choices are unhealthy— meaning we have just a few things to choose that *are* healthy! That should make it easier for us. Find those few things and stick with them!

Americans are getting bigger at an alarming rate! It is worthwhile to try to fix all that is wrong with social security, medicare etc. However, unless we get Americans thinner and healthier, they won't be living long enough to need all of these benefits! It has been estimated by the government, that at the current rate, almost all Americans will be considered overweight by the year 2020! Let's not allow that premonition to come true. Let's get the $150 Billion dollars spent on weight related health problems under control!

I would like to make the first recommendation regarding the food pyramid! We are taught growing up, what the food pyramid is, and how it looks. It has been said that are educational books are 25 years behind. (I'm sure cost has a lot to do with it, although the Internet will be the new form of keeping all teachings up to date, with the latest research, discoveries, and knowledge). I would like to revise it here for you! Stick to the these basics— those few things that make a healthy foundation for life, and you will be successful in all you do!

The pyramid shall now look like this:
The Food Pyramid According to Julia

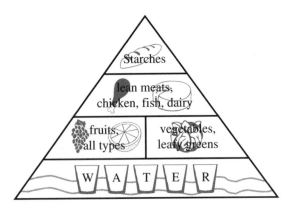

LEVEL I— Your foundation for health
WATER, WATER, WATER

Drink so much water that you begin to feel like Hoover Dam! Initially, you will make frequent trips to the bathroom. This is fine. Your body is getting a good flushing out. I drink so much water in any given day, I require a squeeze bottle next to me and I drink it all day long! If you travel for your job, always bring bottled water along on the flight! I drink a ½ liter prior to landing! Eventually having it with you all the time will be second nature to you!

If I told you that all you had to do was drink a gallon of water a day and you would loose all your weight within a year and keep it off as long as you continued to drink your water; would you? Try me! That is not a license to eat a banana cream pie every night and fill up on water! You have to eat the reasonable way that

I suggest, AND drink your water! I guarantee if you drink 2 liters of water per day, you will have major changes in your health for the better. What?! You want me to tell you the end of the story already, what will happen to you if you do this?..... Where would the diet industry be if all you had to do was drink water. Maybe they're just not telling you, but the changes will be dramatic if you drink the amount I suggest!

I once saw two of the most stunning women at an airport, models I would assume. They each carried a gallon of water and a cup, they were continually drinking water, keeping their perfect figures *perfect*. Little wonder they had such beautiful bodies and complexions! Water is a powerful substance for keeping a good, healthy body.

One final note on water. If you are worried about your community's water, buy bottled or get a water filter for your faucet. Remember, with the quantity you're going to drink everyday, it's as important as the comfort of your bed where at least 25% of your entire life is spent. This should be at least 25% of all that you consume, probably more like 50%! You are 2/3 water, so should be what you consume!

LEVEL II— vitamin and mineral rich
FRUITS AND VEGETABLES

My inclination is to tell you to eat all varieties and as much as you want. That is what I did, it worked for me, but some "expert" might disagree. Make up your mind as to what works for you. Fruit will not make or keep you fat! Mother nature will not be a disappointment for you.

Also, fruits and vegetables are water based items. What this means is that by eating more fruits and vegetables you will be getting additional water in your diet. Of course, being that we are 2/3 water, it is only natural that most of the foods we eat are water based products. This is why fruits and vegetables are used in "juicers." I don't use or recommend using one, because the second important aspect to fruits and vegetables is the fiber content. (In my recipe book, I point out to use a blender instead in order that you still get the fiber.)

A good source of fiber!

Fiber is one of many things we here is missing in our diets, indicated in all the claims of different cereals with high fiber content. The reason our fiber consumption has gotten so low, is because our vegetable and fruit consumption has dropped substantially in the last 20 years! I don't see too many fast food restaurants serving broccoli or spinach. By consuming enough of fruits and vegetables, you can rest assured that your body will respond extremely well! I've never seen someone who was overweight because all they ate was carrots and broccoli. With vegetables, you will get substantial fiber. Human Drano® is what I call them! Vegetables have a way of flushing your system, de-toxing you and cleaning you out! This is probably the most used of all the food groups to me! If I am going to a party, I bring a veggie tray! I graze on veggies all day on one of my binging days (during PMS!) And there's beans, too, to which I sing: "Beans, beans, the magical food, the more you eat the more you lose!!!" — or something like that! One of my snacks during the day was baby carrots. Here are some items to consider:

Fruits:

Avocado (fatty, but high in essential in fats! A great treat every now and then—use cilantro with it to jazz up your chicken breasts!), blackberries, blueberries, cantaloupe, cherries, grapefruit, honeydew, kiwi, peaches, pears, pineapple, plums, raspberries, strawberries, apples, oranges, bananas

Vegetables: Those leafy greens!!

Leafy greens (generally, the darker they are, the higher the vitamin and mineral content), broccoli, carrots, spinach, cauliflower, onion, pickles, zucchini, sauerkraut, snow peas, eggplant, cucumber, mushrooms, summer squash

LEVEL III— building strength
PROTEINS/MEATS

Protein is the what makes up muscles. Put plain and simple, muscles can burn fat! Muscles require more calories to function, so more muscle tone means more calories constantly burning. Therefore, some of your extra fat will be used by the muscles. Too much or too little protein will not allow your system to function optimally. Many experts will tell us that you should consume more carbs than protein, However, make sure that my pyramid is what you follow— meaning you don't want to survive on bread and pasta. You want to eat a small amount of breads, more proteins and then get the rest of your carbos from fruits and vegetables! And, of course, lots of water!

Sources of lean proteins

Meats: beef tenderloin, extra lean ground sirloins, brisket and chuck, chicken breast meat-no skin, pork tenderloin
Dairy: lite cheeses, skim milk, low-fat yogurt, low-fat cottage cheese, egg whites
Protein powders: Great in smoothies! Great as a morning or afternoon meal, although you need a meal with all the food

groups. Use this every now and then, more as a treat. Great to put into the kids shakes! My kids actually ask for smoothies for breakfast now!

Seafood: Many types are good, the light colored tend to be better. Experiment with all types and find those you like!

Turkey: breast with out skin

LEVEL IV— burn fats in a flame of...
STARCHES: Carbohydrates

You want carbs that are high in fiber, and low in sugar and low in starch. Think of an over-starched shirt. You don't want to put that into your body! Not that you would end up stiff, unless of course you visualize 'dead'! That is a real threat of obesity, so perhaps we should scare ourselves a bit!

It has also been said that "fats burn best in a flame of carbohydrates." What this means is that a little carbohydrates before exercising is necessary to start the chemical reaction which gets the fats burning during that exercise. Of course, if you're not going to exercise, then it is obvious you want to limit your intake until you do. Some good source of good carbohydrates are listed here:

Carbohydrates

Oatmeal, OatBran cereal, Shredded wheat, barley; pearl or rolled, buckwheat, Brown rice, Rye crisp crackers, lightly cooked pasta-protein enriched, wheat, taco shells, flour tortilla (look for wheat or variety) if you have to have bread, stick with a bagel-small, wheat bread or a multi-grain!

How our government cannot stress the importance of water in our diets is beyond me! Our bodies are made up of water, without it we die. Yet it isn't even given an honorable mention in a food pyramid! We all need a wake up call. Perhaps it isn't even our fault. We are inundated every where we turn with ads for big sized fast food meals, all you can eat specials, bran muffins (w/ 30 grams of fat), posing as a healthy alternative to a doughnut! How are we to decipher all of this junk in our food!? You must be aware of what you are eating, you must stop yourself before each time you eat and ask yourself, is this really healthy? Will this get me closer to my dreams or further away? The response will be obvious— if it hinders you, put it down! You *can* do this and it *will* become second nature! It is merely being conscience of what you do. Being awakened, if you will.

As a country, we spend billions of dollars on health care for weight related illnesses. If we could all realize the improved quality of life to be had by not putting too much food in our bodies, we would have such a healthy planet!

You don't need me to give you a menu and tell you what to eat at every minute of your day. You know if what you are eating is healthy. You know what to do, just don't delay doing it. YOU need my help in getting yourself motivated to do it, and to do it now! If I could grant you a magic wish, one where you could wake up tomorrow morning in a thin body, or a wish that you would stay the same, would you choose to be thin? We all want to be "in shape," we just don't always want to work at it. It is the fact that it requires some work and the results take time to see. That is what keeps us from getting started.

Realize that your dreams and goals really are just a day away. Each day believing "today I will live my dreams," you will be a day away everyday. Change will soon take place, and then you will set your sites on higher goals, soon after reaching them, pushing you toward your full potential!!

Preparing Mentally

I want to help you see that you must get serious about your health, right now, today, this very minute! WHY?— For your health, for the quality of your life, for your self esteem, for your family, and even for your sex life, the list goes on and on! I promise you that every aspect of your life will be improved once you conquer that which is holding you back. For me it was my inability to lose weight, and overcoming the mental block that was keeping me from getting started. Since over coming it, I know that I am a better mother, community member, parishioner, friend, volunteer, worker and partner (at the risk of giving the ending away, a better wife, too!)

What is it that is causing your mental block? Is it a lack of *reason* for wanting to lose weight? Are you in a relationship where you are sabotaging yourself as punishment like I was? Or is it something from childhood that has you mentally conditioned? Look inside to find what has kept you from making the decision to reach your goals. Maybe you just need a healthy addiction like exercise rather than food— *replacing a bad addiction with a good one.* Or quite possibly, you just need to begin loving yourself in a way that delays gratification. After all, I know I used food to make me feel good, and all the while it was hiding the pain. The real pain was that I was not happy with me as a person. That may or may not be yours. But look at yourself and what will happen if you don't change.

If what I say is true, what do you have to lose by doing it, what do you have to gain? There is a method of evaluating something called—-doing a 'Ben Franklin.' In doing this, you write down Pros and Cons of the decision you need to make. On a piece of paper make a line down the middle, then list your pros and cons of losing weight. Or you could look at it as the pros and cons of NOT losing weight. (For that matter, you can do the pros and cons of not making the decision to change. That way, this can be used in many different areas of your life!) Here are mine:

PROS	CONS
Increased health	declining health
More energy	less energy
Buy clothes at more places	hard to find clothes
Feel more attractive	feel less attractive
Save money on food	waste money on food
More interest from men	men less interested
Healthier sex life	Maybe no sex life at all
Better attitude toward all	depression & anxiety
Confident, take more chances	live in fear
More time for others	only think of myself
Able to earn more money	not as productive
Increased longevity	may have early death
Can be active for years	may never be active
Tasks not limited	may not fit into a chair
Can make more friends	may lose friends
Will feel free	will feel trapped inside
Will smile more often	may not smile again
Can help change the world	not as good to others
Able to fulfill dreams	Less likely to reach
Can be proud of who I am	Will be ashamed
Will die with a smile	Will be dead before I die

These are things that I thought of. If you can relate to any of the above, take time to really picture yourself— on both sides, so you not only feel the pleasure that will come with the pros, but the pain that will come with the cons. Remember, this is your list and your life! Don't waste any more time! In fact, that should be at the top of your list— more available productive and active time, the other side being wasted time!!

Basic Principles for Success

The big picture as to what caused me to get on the right track towards fitness and health was realizing that my life was out of my control. I wanted it back, my life and the control. Sure, I wanted to lose weight, and I blamed my obesity for a lot of my ills, but it was more than that. There are different reasons for different people, but I knew that I couldn't rely on someone else for my happiness any longer. I wasn't happy when I tried that, it didn't work. It was time to try something new! It all had to start with me. And **it all has to start with you!**

I believe that this is a realization we all must have to get us on the right track for life. Once you realize that your decisions are the key to moving you in the right direction, you will never want to go back to the old way of life again. The pride and sense of self that you get from actually accomplishing the objectives that you set for yourself is amazing, it is life changing! Start enjoying a good diet, including vitamins, minerals and supplements to aid in supporting a healthy metabolism. Ensure your body gets the proper nutrients to function efficiently and promote weight loss. Incorporate exercising, renewing old interests, getting out, trying new things... The more that you do these things, your old image will become a distant, memory which is no longer painful, and you'll begin creating new happy memories!

I decided that it was time **get rid of what I was mostly made of... FAT!** The human body is not meant to carry a lot of extra useless tissue, it's just insulation it believes it needs from the extra consumption. What does that mean? It means lose weight or the weight will continue to stress your body and it will break down. Lose weight or the vehicle that houses your soul will stop working. Unlike cars, you can't trade your body in on a newer, sleeker or racier model! But you can, thank God, remodel the one you have!

Obesity is the second leading cause of preventable death in our country. According to the National Research Council for Health, 35% of Americans are obese, that breaks down to 1 in 3 of us! If it is not the persons sitting to the left or right of you, it is YOU!! You may be at risk of dying well before your time if this is true. Not a pleasant thought!

So what choices did I make to get from 265+ lbs. down to the 135 pounds that I am

My simple choices

today? Knowing my body weight was a direct result of the eating decisions I had made, I decided to *change one point...* eat less fattening foods. **I cut out the fat!** It was that simple. Don't worry, I didn't bring you this far to tell you what you probably already knew...eat less fat! Although I will stress that this is very key to losing weight, it isn't everything! You have to get the big picture right! What led me to make this change was **the deeper, more meaningful life I wanted to create for myself.**

You must first change the way you *think* about food. I mentioned children and your role in what they eat. I am concerned with the high numbers of children put on major drugs like Ritalin® each year. I wonder if we as parents wouldn't see these problems, along with the epidemic of childhood obesity, drastically decrease in number if we would only eliminate the sugar filled cereals, high sugar drinks and the fattening snacks we feed our children— giving them instead vitamins and well rounded meals, as well as limiting the amount of time each day that our children watch tv or play video games! **"Garbage in equals garbage out"** comes to mind. You are what you eat, and your body will resemble your activity level. Lead the life of an athlete, you will be built like one; lounge about, you will look like you do!

So think of food as a source of energy for strength and stamina— physically as well as mentally and spiritually! If your not going to use it for one of these three, then don't eat it!

**Making smart,
simple choices**

Begin by making smart choices about what you eat. To help you make those smart choices, I am including a grocery list of suggested foods. This list appears at the end of the book. I would suggest tearing it out and carrying it with you. It is a guide with some suggestions, add more of what you like as well but avoid the junk aisles. Ultimately, you must decide what foods you will eat and enjoy. The goal is eating healthy foods that you like so that you will stick with it! I don't want you following a rigid eating plan that I set for you, only to have you decide you don't like the foods I recommend, resulting in you throwing the whole book out in the trash feeling denied of your chance!

There are so many choices that are available to you, healthy choices as well as unhealthy. The choice has to be yours. You have to decide to eat the fruits, vegetables and lean meats rather than the pastries, cookies, fried foods and fatty sauces—   not just for the next few days, weeks or months, but forever! **The principle here is to be in control, and having enough reasons "why" you want to be in control.** You must make these choices consistently and forever. It is **never** acceptable to gorge yourself on fat, or you will be that— FAT!! Even the people who are thin have no need to eat fat laden food! We all have the same hearts, arteries, etc....thin or fat, your body can't function at it's optimal level fueled with unhealthy food!

Taking Control of Life!

It comes down to this: **KEEP IT SMART AND SIMPLE** (K.I.S.S.)   You   must   set

The K.I.S.S. system

yourself up for success, not doom yourself to defeat as every diet does by the mere fact that it is a diet! It is not a "program," a "regimen," a "prescription," a "*diet!*" All things that assume there is a beginning, and an end— something that you have to start, stay on, and consider it wrong when you eat unhealthy. After all, isn't it wrong to do drugs, not just because they are illegal, but because they will do damage to your body? How about a cheese cake? It's not now, nor will ever be a healthy option for fueling your body! (Unless your stranded on a desert island with only that to eat)! Find the things that are healthy and taste good, and make them your only choices: Keeping things smart and simple!

When I started changing my eating habits, this was what I ate for a typical day for me: I started my day with bran cereal. Initially, I ate a huge bowlful with a touch of sugar. I was hungry! If 11 p.m. rolled around and I felt hungry, I'd have another bowl. Eventually, my appetite died down, and yours will too. The human Drano® effect that it had made me want to eat less of it too! In the beginning, I ate the quantity I needed to be satisfied, making certain that I made only healthy choices for what I ate. I didn't concern myself with the amount of food as much as I did the content of the food itself.

To manage between-meal munchies at work, I kept a bag of baby carrots next to my desk. I know myself and I am a nibbler. Stress makes me eat, nervousness makes me eat. Knowing this about myself allowed me to plan for it. I grazed all day on my carrots or other fruits and vegetables I would bring to the office! I remember eating so many carrots in one day that, while on my way home, I looked in the rear view mirror and saw that my teeth were orange! Actually orange! Thank goodness, after a quick round with my toothbrush they were once again pearly white! Otherwise, given my hot temper at the time, I would have resigned to a sweet.

An occasional sweet tooth!

For sweet-tooth emergencies, I kept another stash in my desk—Starburst™. If my sweet tooth beckoned, I could answer in a controlled manner... No pastry binges, nor a half-gallon lite ice cream. A Starburst™ or two, with just a few calories, and I felt satisfied— not denied. I highly recommend the green wrapped banana mango flavor! If the chocolate monster came to call, a Hershey's Kiss™ helped curb my sweet tooth and added only a few calories and only a gram of fat. I kept them in the freezer, they were quite satisfying for the former ice cream addict that I was! Far better than a dozen creme-filled doughnuts! I have a weakness for chocolate chip cookies, I would be lying if I said I didn't have one or two occasionally as well. Before, I was putting such large amounts of food into my body. Once I stopped doing that— stopped the half gallon of ice cream a night, etc...having a few normal treats— then once in a great while having a treat didn't hinder me losing weight and the absence of the vast amounts of fatty foods made losing weight inevitable! Also, the occasional treat kept me from needing to binge, so keeping those desires in check!

The way I look at it, everyday life has its stresses. Traffic tickets(I've had my share!), highway pileups, running late for work, meeting deadlines, bills, arranging schedules with your partner, meeting the needs of your kids, and on and on— why add to that by dieting and dumping on yourself if you stray from the rigid regime? Not to mention good, healthy eating habits allow you to get through the stresses *much* easier. Life is too short for self-inflicted punishment! Whether you are thin or obese, young or old, your body can't operate efficiently with "garbage" food!

A mother called me recently about her 18 year old daughter who weighs close to 300 pounds. The woman was distraught. She had taken her daughter to medical doctors who pronounced the girl healthy, and nothing medically wrong with her. He declared that she had the "fat gene" and that nothing could be done. That is how a medical doctor left it! Nothing could be done? A fat gene? The research that I have read tells me that very few obese people have a genetic predisposition to it, it is merely an excuse given, not to mention there are still many things that can be done to increase the **quality** of her life! The mother went on to tell me that no one else in the family is overweight, and that the daughter eats all the same food they do— fast food, fries, Mexican dishes, dessert, yet she keeps getting bigger and they don't!

The problem was clear to me— the rest of the family had a problem! Against all odds, they weren't gaining weight (at least, not yet!). With a diet like she mentioned they should all weigh 300 pounds! I told her that none of them, much less someone looking to lose weight needed to eat this way! Here is an example where the visible sign of unhealthy eating was not present— that is, they weren't overweight. This doesn't imply that they *are* healthy. Cancer many times does not show symptoms until the person is within days of death! In other words, eating unhealthy has more effects on you than what may or may not be showing!

Environmentalists got us to quit using leaded gas for reasons related to the environment and our health— for God's sake quit eating 'leaded' food and allow your body to run better!! It is ridiculous that we are so hypocritical as to make changes for the good of environment, yet we continue to be gorge ourselves into being an obese society. We are cutting years off our lives— years we won't have to live in the cleaner world that the unleaded fuel is facilitating. The local fast food restaurants are super-sizing® their meals, as though they weren't caloric enough, now you can get enough calories to sustain a family of four in one person's "serving." It is like a drug pusher, avoiding telling his customers that what he is selling them is harmful to their health, and instead offering them bigger, better, more enticing deals to lure the addict back again and again!

As you start to change your habits, remember something very important that a person very dear to me reminded me,

"If a little is good, it doesn't mean more is better!"

This is a good thought to keep in mind. With all the buffets and all-you-can-eat restaurants, we have taken food to an addiction worse than any drug ever made. Keep the portions small, no matter what it is. It would be like exercising the first time and saying "well, if 30 minutes are good, 4 hour must be better." Now you subject yourself to possible injury.

Make the decision to cut out the fat, the overly processed foods, things with ingredients that have no end to their shelf life, and decide to eat healthy from this moment on, forever!! Can you have a cookie every now and then? Sure. Why buy packaged, processed and chemically enhanced cookies, though. If you have to have a cookie, get a fresh bakery cookie or better yet make some with your kids, then give them away!! The local police will love you if you drop off a fresh batch of cookies! You won't be tempted to eat them and the officers might think twice before giving you a ticket if they see you speeding (while on your way to your workout?!).

Experiment in your kitchen with new seasonings and spices. I use a lot of fresh basil and cilantro in my cooking, even mint. They add so much flavor to food and few or no calories! Make healthy food taste good. This isn't a prison, you can get creative, you just need to be aware and smart about your choices! Keep things smart and simple.

SUPPLEMENTS

Educate yourself as to the advances in weight-loss-enhancing supplements and vitamins. Under **"The once dreaded: Exercise"** section in a few pages, I discuss a couple of excellent products. You will find products able to help not only your weight loss, but your health in general. I am rarely ill since losing the weight that I did. I wonder if it is that fact alone or a combination of the healthy foods I eat and the wonderful vitamins and supplements that I use! I like to think it is a combination of good physical health (nutrition and exercise), mental health (attitude), as well as spiritual.

I recommend you ask your medical doctor or chiropractor what vitamins and supplements they would recommend for you and encourage you take them religiously. If you have trouble getting out, Internet sites or cable shopping channels, such as QVC, they can ship your supplements directly to your door every month!

There really are no excuses, today's technology makes life easier, utilize it! Spend your time taking care of yourself! There are products on the market that can help to maintain a healthy metabolism, such as Chromium Picolinate. Even Chitosan based products that actually binds to the fat in that occasional cookie so your body doesn't absorb any new fat! I personally think that discovery deserves a Nobel Prize! Think of the mass of humanity that is going to serve!! *Even still, there will be people who won't take such a product because deep down they don't really desire to better themselves.*

Vitamins and minerals help every cell in your body function more effectively! Just keep my basic rule in mind, "if a little is good, it doesn't mean that more is better!" Use your basic smarts. Even the best fat binding product or metabolism booster is not a license to overeat— but great assistance in helping you achieve a goal! They can also be great tools to help support your body's health and metabolism, and even suppress eating binges! Taking vitamins and minerals does not negate the need to fuel your body with a variety of fruits, vegetables and proteins. Ultimately, the only way to lose weight and keep it off forever is for you to make the decision everyday that you are in charge of what goes into your body. The decision is yours to make, not that of the food you eat!

GETTING STARTED

Start today by being your best friend. You wouldn't tie up your best friend and insist he or she eat a gallon of ice cream, would you? Then, why do it to yourself? Why do that which seems to be your downfall, why set yourself up for failure? Eat healthy 90-95 percent of the time and you'll be within the boundaries of healthy eating. Then, if you absolutely have to eat a chocolate chip cookie, eat one. Of course, be sure to ask yourself if you really have to have one. Most of the time I'm sure you will find the answer to be no, but still it won't ruin your weight loss or make you gain weight. The key is: stop at one. Treat your body like a temple; feed it wonderful, healthy food. I completely swore off the ice cream! To this day, I won't eat it, and it isn't difficult any more, but it wasn't easy at first. I did crave it, but I convinced myself that it was to blame for my unhappiness. I made myself come to hate it!

See for yourself how much damage the food of choice is to your body—leave some ice cream in a dish in the sink and come back to it hours later. Look at how it appears now! It is a sticky glob of fat! Totally gross! If bread is your weakness, add some water to a bowl, and put the bread in it. Look at it hours later, it almost resembles glue! You won't want that junk in your body, trust me! Even now, I can't eat it, I won't eat it; for I never want to return to the place I was at in life!

Studies show that if you repeat an action everyday for 21 days, it becomes a habit. Through my own experience, it is now my opinion that after you eat this way for three weeks, it too becomes habit. Your body and mind will actually crave this healthy food.

Imagine, three weeks out of your entire life, just to form the good, healthy habits that will lead to a lifetime of health, happiness, and joy! Twenty-one days out of an average life expectancy of 76 years, is .0757% of the total days you will probably live. To put it another way, that's 21 days out of 27,740 total days. Not many to make life-changing habits for the better— that will last forever!

To further help establish the habit and take your mind off food, I recommend that you find a healthy, filling item or meal and eat that for lunch every day. This will keep things simple and smart. For variety, you may want to switch to a new item each week. I ate my Veggie Sandwich (found in the back pages) almost everyday for seven months! It's true, and I am proof that it works. Here's why: it helps **take your mind off food— what to eat, how to prepare it, how much to eat— giving you time and energy to focus on other things.**

> **Find other things in life!**

You don't want to wrap yourself up in the hassles of trying to lose weight. Make the decisions now, and leave it at that for months to come. This way you can do other things with your time and energy than worry about food! It is boring, sure, but it is just food! It really isn't intended to be the mainstay of our thoughts— it is fuel for your body, period. Take the importance in your life away from food, and take back the control! We have to eat to live, don't live to eat!

For example, by reading a good book, magazine or newspaper, it can help you put your mind on something else. Read about what some Hollywood stars, or what members of your own community are doing. Things that you would like to be doing, that you will do, given the road you're now on! The important component is that you're eating healthy food, and the pounds are falling off without having to focus on losing weight all the time.

Throughout my weight loss, it was easiest to bring my week's worth of groceries into the office on Monday. That way I didn't have to think about lunch, what I'd eat, where to go get it, whether I'd have enough, etc. Before adopting this simple routine, I used to spend so much time thinking about what I would eat, would it be healthy, etc!! Its easy to overeat if you need to think about food all the time! If it consumes your mind, then it will consume your actions as well!

In the past, I would start thinking about lunch at 10:00, where I would go, what I would

Ah! Too many decisions!!

order. Thinking "Should I get Chinese food, fried rice, no MSG? Right, that would be a good choice. No, that is oily, perhaps I should go to the salad bar. I won't get the egg, meat or cheese. Low fat dressing...yeah, that would work. Oh, I know, I will get a veggie pizza delivered to me here, that way I can stay and work through lunch. And I'm feeling pretty good today, add a little extra cheese." Its no wonder I couldn't lose weight!

Looking back I can see now why I always believed I was dieting and eating healthy, because I put so much thought and effort into it! If effort meant anything, I would have been thin long before! Once I quit dwelling on what I would eat, life got a lot easier! At 11:30 a.m. each day, I'd go to the kitchen in my office and make my sandwich and eat— simple process without a great deal of thought required. The guys at work nicknamed my lunch staple (Veggie Sandwich) the "stinky sandwich" because, when heated in the microwave, the broccoli and Swiss cheese on it emitted a strong odor. Smelly, maybe, but it sure tasted great—and still does! My Veggie Sandwich is a standard lunch for me—one I eat at least once a week!

Another thing that I did might be fun for you too. I recruited others in my office who were interested in healthy eating and formed a "fat-free lunch club." Each day, one person was responsible for bringing enough lunch to feed themselves as well as the others in the group! It was a lot of fun and enabled me to try new recipes and get to know my co-workers better.

Dinner was easy— that wasn't the time of day that I was the hungriest. Worn out after a long day, then rushing to cook for everyone else, I didn't have the appetite I did at other times throughout the day. Usually, I'd have a serving of the vegetables and fruit I had prepared for my kids, adding brown rice or pasta. Once or twice a week I splurged on a fresh veggie pizza (most large supermarkets have one they make fresh daily), with little to no cheese!

A great food item that I recently discovered and I would highly recommend is Gardenburger® veggie patties. If you are like me and love the whole hamburger "experience," these are for you! They are meatless patties, low in fat, all natural, and they have a bunch of great flavors— my favorites are the Savory Mushroom and the Veggie Medley flavors. (You should be able to find them in the frozen section of most grocery stores!)

In Style!

On the weekends, something I loved to do was to make a tray of grapes, lite crackers, some good paté and leave it around to nibble, like at a cocktail party! I even put my sparkling water in a crystal wine glass! Just because I was alone didn't mean I couldn't do it in style! Setting a mood made me feel that I was treating myself to the best natural substances for my body—in style! If you place fresh flowers on your table, use pretty dishes, play some classical music while you dine. It will bring up your level of appreciation for treating yourself well— not just shoveling food down! The atmosphere should be more the focus and more enjoyable than the food!

Prepare an evening for the entire family. Start with a salad with leafy greens, great vegetables, a low calorie dressing, perhaps a slice of multi-grain bakery bread, and a large glass of iced tea or water. While giving thanks, let everyone take turns saying what they are thankful for about their day. Listen to what made everyone's day special, or if you are alone, reflect on what gifts you had that day, and those to look forward to. Focus on spending "quality time" with your loved ones. It is a great time for really finding out what goes on in your kids lives! Move onto the next course— lean meat, steamed vegetables, a small potato perhaps.

After dinner, enjoy fresh seasonal fruit, and *occasionally* have a treat, maybe angel food cake or pumpkin pie, (although I do recommend that if you eat any treats, you do so in the middle of the day, so you have the rest of the day to burn it off!). Healthy menus like these are great, not only for you, but for your family, too. I love when women tell me they can't make a "healthy" meal because they have to cook for their whole family, not just themselves. I have before said the exact same comment!

Stop and think about that comment, do only *you* deserve to eat healthy? Are your children or your

Family cooking!

spouse any less deserving of healthy bodies and a longer life? Just think, everyone will benefit from your healthy lifestyle and the new you! Plus, you'll bestow healthy eating habits in your children that will carry with them through life. Will they complain and fight you initially when you introduce grilled chicken instead of nuggets fried in lard? Of course! But they also fight about bed time, tooth brushing and getting shots! You wouldn't back down from your insistence on these vital points, now would you?

You may have gotten my cookbook along with this book. In it, I try to include easy recipes—those that are healthy and don't take a lot of time. This keeps the focus away from food! Another cookbook that I would recommend is *Looneyspoons,* written by two sisters from Canada. Just remember, "if a little is good, more isn't better." They have some great family friendly recipes that you can even involve the kids in preparing! After a few weeks of meals together, it will be much more about being together as a family, than about the food you are eating. It will be so "Norman Rockwell" you won't believe it!

The recipes included in the back pages are satisfying, taste great and have a low fat content. They truly were the staples of my weight loss. I particularly love the pasta dish with fresh vegetables and Dijon mustard. If too much times goes by and I haven't eaten this dish, I use it again. I continue to eat these foods because, as I've told you from the start, this is NOT a diet— *it's a lifestyle*!!

Many people have asked me for more recipes, even though I am not known for my culinary flare. I like simple, easy to make and quick, healthy meals. I think that I am a good cook, just not too fancy. So I did go through some recipes that were used during my weight loss, and those that I use today. I added a few that are special occasion meals, but for the most part all are very simple and smart recipes. **The recipe book is available through a couple of sources. It is called: "Take-Control Recipes."** Bear in mind that my overall philosophy is that food isn't the focus of our lives— it is just the necessary fuel, not to be an addictive pleasure!

My short recipe book has focused on the same philosophy— tasty and satisfying, but not too time consuming to prepare. You need to begin to derive pleasure out of living *life* to it's fullest, not making your belly it's fullest! It must be a lifelong lifestyle change you make that will take the weight off and keep it off permanently. Your body will be able to efficiently burn the healthier foods you will be eating and you will soon become your ideal weight. With simple changes and nothing drastic or severe!

I can say that with simple eating habits, I was able to take my mind off of eating and focus on other things. This message causes me to reflect on another point. When so many areas of my life suffered from my being overweight, either directly or indirectly, I knew that I needed to change many things. So first it was a matter of needing to simplify my eating habits because I needed time and energy to pull other areas of my life together. Then, only later did I realize that this was the same thinking that allowed me to enjoy my life— I was focusing on **IT** *rather than pleasing myself with food! I think you will find the same to be true!*

The once-dreaded: EXERCISE!

One of the things I regret I did not do for the first six months of my new lifestyle, is exercise.   I lost a lot of weight without exercise, so I know that just eating right can make huge changes to your body. However, with exercise, it is likely that I would have lost weight even more quickly, and I'll always wonder if the loose sagging skin I was left with would have shrunk naturally (or sooner) had I started a program initially.   Either way, today I am working out and have been since I lost the weight.

My recommendation is to get active— today! Don't wait until you feel thin enough to go to the gym. Go now, and reap the benefits from working out.   Your progress will be exponential compared to not exercising at all.   Everyone is there for the same reason and will respect your desire to improve your body.   You'll be surprised at how supportive others will be of your program. There is always someone at the gym or aerobics class ready to give you a compliment or applaud your efforts, as should you— as we're all in this together.

I was telling this to a group of women recently and they didn't believe that the spandex set at the gym truly cared about them. I assured them that it was not true and that if no one had yet approached them with a kind word of encouragement, it is simply that they don't want to make them self conscience! I am sure of that! I want to go up and offer encouragement to some of my fellow step classmates, but I stop myself and remember how I felt and I know I would have doubted someone's sincerity. So I applaud my classmates efforts silently!

Taking Control of Life!

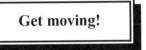

Get moving!

If right now you are large and having trouble moving about, realize that ANY exercise is better than none. The more often you do it, the easier it will get. There are some exercise videos available that may assist you with an at-home program if you elect to do so. Remember to stay within your limit starting out if you don't already.

Find what exercise you enjoy and do it! Believe me or not, eventually you too can become one of those people addicted to working out! Be smart when you are just getting started. One of the biggest mistakes that people make is they pledge to do an hour on the treadmill everyday until they are thin! While an hour would be great, it is not realistic to think that you could do this your first week! Gradually build up to an hour! Start with 20 minutes (even 5 minutes!), 3 times a week— *that* won't "kill" you! You won't be sore in the morning and you won't burn out before you even get going!! If you do a moderate amount of everything healthy— eating healthy, exercising, being active, etc.— it will add up to a whole lot of healthy actions!

Get a workout partner

As you go through these changes in your life, it helps to find a partner that desires to improve upon their body, in order that you can help motivate each other. Or, perhaps there is someone you know who has already achieved their goal and can be a true source of mental support. We all need that support system to buck us up when we start to fall. I'd love to be the support system to help you through that.

I never thought I would, but here I am as living proof! I

know the instructors by name, I have friends in the classes and I love watching each change my body makes as it continues week after week to improve! It is a challenge now to see at age 36, what level of fitness I can get my body to! I held my weight at 146 lbs., for almost 3 years.

Working out 5 times a week and eating healthy (I would be lying if I didn't admit to the occasional chocolate chip cookie!), I had reached a new plateau. I decided to find a natural supplement to help me reach my desired goal. During most of my 120 pound loss, I used a couple of different products consistently. I decided to look for a product that contained these, while also researching what others were out there.

A great weight loss supplement!

I came across a product relatively new to an industry with literally thousands of natural weight loss supplements out there. In fact, one particular product caught my attention after thoroughly investigating many different ones. After looking at many other products, I decided to use this Chitosan based product that binds to the fat in foods eaten, so you don't absorb the fat into your body. Combined with an appetite suppressant I used in the morning, the results have been magnificent. And for those women I speak with who have also tried it, their results have been overwhelming! I have been *able to lose 10 more pounds in less than 3 months— after being on a plateau for more than 2 years!*

I truly believe that there are other benefits than the "physiological" ones with any product. By taking a supplement as these every day, you not only are providing your body with an action that will help with your weight loss (or maintenance), but the "psychological" element is also present. Just taking a supplement each day reminds you that your are on a healthy road, making healthy decisions. *That* itself increases your awareness and realization, of the fact that your are moving toward your goals. Beneath the 10 pounds I was holding during my 2 year plateau, I was building some impressive muscle tone, and now it is now beginning to show! I am love this stuff! Marie Antoinette could be a great spokesperson: "have your cake and eat it, too!"

Be sure that you follow the directions suggested, and please, be consistent with your use of them, as with all of the recommendations I give you here. By taking just one action each day, you will make very significant changes in no time!

A cute story that I will share with you is the "Eat the Cake"story. An 87-year old woman refused to eat her birthday cake for fear it was too caloric and would raise her cholesterol level. She died 2 weeks later! Isn't life too short to pass up **birthday** *cake? You'll need to if you're* **dieting!** *But if your living healthy and exercising, you can rest assured that this is just apart of the day's celebration—not a food celebration. You can celebrate life! Knowing that you will be burning more calories with exercise than any cake would ever put on.. This is the chance for you to erase your past behaviors and create a new life for yourself! Get off the sidelines and start playing in the game!*

I think about one complaint that I got from the first edition of my book. The woman

One reader's response

told me she was going to use the book to level out an uneven dresser, that was all it would ever do to help her! Did she ever sound like the old unhappy me. I remember my attitude that if you couldn't promise to make me thin, I wouldn't dare look at myself as the potential problem source! I was thinking how I wanted to change her attitude to focus on the positive, but it is something that will only come from within.

I try to respond to everyone that contacts me, because it is very fulfilling to see someone turn their life around. I am totally committed to helping you achieve your goals and dreams! Without a doubt this whole experience has been one of the most incredible things that has ever happened to me in my life. Being a mother, falling in love, and helping others better their lives— it doesn't get any better! It would give me great inspiration to hear your success story! E-mail me and let me know how *you're* doing!

STICK WITH IT!

OK, now that you're ready to live healthy and smart, and be active, let's emphasize another important point. KEEP WITH IT! It won't happen overnight. It took me a year to lose 95 pounds. A few more months for a total of 125 to come off. Now after a few years, I am just about my ideal weight at 136 lbs. (5' 7" tall). In the big picture of life, that's not long at all! At the time, it did seem like forever. Remember our earlier calculations? How does 1 year out of 74 sound? It will go by FAST!

I want you to know that I understand your feeling of despair, those thoughts of "it just won't happen for me!" It will, but it does take time! I became very conscious of myself, always evaluating each part of my body every step of the way. The changes, while gradual, were amazing to me— I marveled each time I could tell a big difference in my appearance! The milestones reached along the way to thinness were great motivation. I remember thinking after my first 10 pounds— "Wow, depression works for me!" Then people started to notice and complimenting me. I began to think, "I *do* look better; this shirt *is* a bit looser!"

It is that kind of positive reinforcement that kept me going, so I wouldn't revert to my old unhealthy habits. To be honest with you, those compliments still to this day provide a certain amount of motivation. It is a lot nicer to get whistled at by a passing car than have someone call me Barney! I will admit I am flattered by the attention— the few times it has happened though, I'm looking around to see where the pretty girl is!— couldn't be me?!

The best reinforcement came from within me. Honestly, all the comments from others were nice and boosted my ego, but the pride that I felt for making another step in the right direction was better! Once discounting everything I did, now I feel my self worth has been created by knowing that I can make a contribution to others, each day. I feel now a sense of duty and commitment to keeping my standards high, and helping you raise yours, in order that you may meet your goals!

I didn't feel like I was successful or worthy of high self-esteem merely because I was overweight! Being fat doesn't negate your value as a human being, but it may significantly limit the potential you have for yourself and for others! Start beaming with internal pride every time you treadmill for 20 minutes, or pass on the office donuts! Your smile and aura will shine!

LOOKING BACK

Some people evaluate my weight loss story saying, 'Sure you lost the weight because of the divorce.' Forget the fact that I lost a great deal of weight prior to separating! No, the Julia I was then would eat her way out of a funk. I took what was to say the least, an emotionally very low point in my life and chose to better myself. It was a compilation of many things that gave me the motivation to change. But the decision and commitment were the keys to getting on the road. I created a better life for my children and for myself. I feel that now I am doing my part to make the world a better place!

I know people who, after an extra-marital affair was disclosed, have let the misfortune in their lives consume them. They allow their feelings of devastation to cloud over their lives and often funnel their energies into nonproductive channels. I didn't fall apart, but instead took charge of my life. I had spent years allowing the negative in my life to rule my actions, making me a very negative person. When I truly believed that couldn't get any worse, I knew I needed to change. There was nowhere to go but up!

We all need something to jump start our engines, but we have to supply our own fuel. You can be your own energy. In this way there is no better feeling on earth than to face those that have hurt you, hold your head up high and say, "Look at me now. I'm a survivor. I'm strong and I love me!" Hard to imagine feeling that way, but you will! You'll become a larger *being* than you ever were!

Look around at the world, who accomplishes more in life- - those "weighed" down by too much food in their bodies, or those who are fit and leading active lives? Which do you want to be, sedentary or active?

In speaking with people wherever I go, one question that I am often asked, is "What does your ex think of your weight loss and success?" Initially, I don't think he thought anything of my writing a book, or my goals. But I can only speculate by his behavior that he feels like he missed out on a very special part of what happened to me, and who I am today! Of course, I say this not knowing for sure, but I also feel I wouldn't be the person I am now without the shakeup that occurred.

There are two people in a relationship. And while he strayed, I was the one who quit caring about myself. In his own way, he is proud of me and happy for the life that I have made for myself and for the children. He is a happier person now, too. Negative energy causes everyone it touches harm. Eliminating it in my life, we have all thrived. He has still at times called me a name, but I look past those comments and rejoice in the fact that I am not living in the past. A comment like that now falls on deaf ears. It is a neither true, nor effective any longer to reduce the happiness and joy in my life! Today, we are virtually strangers who happen to share two children. I was a very negative person during the last years we were together, and know that the mind is a very powerful thing! Control what you think enables happiness!

What should I do?

An overweight reader asked me if she should leave her husband. All of her friends say he's a great guy, but she feels they have grown apart. My advice.....focus on improving yourself, and losing the weight along with any negative thoughts. Even getting into counseling to do her best to save her marriage. Relationships and how we deal with them are a big part of who we are. Although, making every attempt to salvage a relationship through communication is and always should be the first option, changing a person that may be very negative is not *always* possible. If you are going to be a happy, healthy, and productive person in life, **being around a similar type of person(s) is the going to be the healthiest way to live!** And sometimes you have to make some hard decisions to do that.

*If you have an older car and are tired of it, then you go out and test drive a new one, the old one will never seem as nice again. If you stopped and thought about your old car, and how reliable it is, perhaps you could give it a bit of attention, clean it up and it would be fine for quite some time to come. Trading in a spouse shouldn't be the option that it has become. It doesn't foster the growth in a relationship or future ones. And that **is** necessary for a happy existence with all people.*

I will never know if our marriage could have been saved, by the time I got myself together, he was long gone emotionally. It happened, I won't say it was all his fault. I know that only I can be responsible for my thoughts and actions. He is now remarried. But I do owe her some thanks. Without her intrusion into my life, I might never have '*awoken the diet within*' me! I might still be a negative, overweight, crabby person wallowing around in self-pity. For that awakening, I thank her. For committing adultery for 2½ years with a married man, well, I know she'll have Someone else to answer to.

That is my personal saga— what relevance does it have to you and your life? In my first book, many readers told me they got the impression that I found out about the betrayal, got divorced and *then* lost weight while holed up in some massive depressive state. As you have read, that wasn't the case. I managed to find the time, energy and determination to change myself, to lose weight and to move ahead, all while my "home" continued to cave in around me. I held it together by taking back the control in my life. Then I was able to rebuild my life and make it better than it ever was! I am not requesting nor deserving of martyr status. I did what had to be done, the alternative would have turned out worse than what my life had been for those past few years.

A ray of hope!

I share with you the intimate and sad details in my life to show you a light, a ray of hope. No matter what you are dealing with, you can see that change is at hand! You are in control and you can come out on top if that is what you decide you are going to do and accepting nothing less than that from yourself! Losing weight is a by-product of self betterment! Self-improvement through self-motivation will certainly make your waist line thinner, and it will not stop there— it truly will improve every aspect of your life!

You may know the story of Pandora's box. She was sent to earth with every human virtue in a sacred box, and was told never to open it. The curiosity got the best of her and she opened the box, letting out all of the virtues....but closing it just in time...***before HOPE was let out! Hence, "there is always HOPE!" Don't give up!***

ACCEPTING CHANGE

Making healthier eating choices, drinking a lot of water, taking vitamins and supplements appropriate to my body type, and making steps to rebuild my damaged self esteem, I began to really believe I was getting somewhere. I have often said I should call my plan the "Vanity Diet." For some, putting emphasis on your physical appearance is vain and self absorbed. I will not argue that point. However, the alternative is not acceptable to me. I had let myself go too far in the other direction. I quit caring how I looked and what I ate. That in turn made me obese, hurt my health and decreased my longevity, as well as giving me a pretty nasty disposition! Getting back in touch with my femininity and caring about my outward appearance, did so much more than make me look better— it made me live better as well!

> **Is it OK to be.. or not..?**

Health issues aside, some people have made the argument that being overweight is not a bad thing, as long as you are happy being who you are. I will state that although this may be true, we are judged by are actions. And if being overweight is any reflection of what actions we have chosen in the past, then there may be a good argument against that statement. There, of course, are always exceptions to the rule. I wasn't the exception and have spoken with many who aren't either.

Weight loss through these basic principles is a synergistic process. The better you look, the better you feel. The more you consume healthy foods, the better your body will feel and look. This reinforces your positive attitude. People begin to notice that something is different about you. You feel great, and soon you'll crave only healthy foods. Your body's response becomes the best motivation for which you could ask! Add a little exercise to get those endorphins flowing and soon, there will be no stopping you!

Time for new clothes?

Before you know it, none of your old clothes will fit. Now, financially, maybe that's not so good, but for motivation sake... watch out! Unfortunately, a new wardrobe will cost money. So, hey—get a sewing machine or borrow one from a friend and run a big seam up the back of all your clothes as they start to bag on you. I realize that it may not be in the best professional taste to have a three-inch seam down the back of your dress, but it will make you so proud of yourself and your weight loss. I wore those seams like medals! I showed everyone and proudly told them, "Look, I had to take this in three inches!" Keep doing it until you reach your goal. Make new clothes your reward for each new goal reached.

Thrift shops are another good alternative. You can purchase inexpensive skirts, blouses, slacks, and sweaters that can be donated back when you're ready to buy clothes in your "ideal" size. Once you get going on the changes I've suggested, the pounds will melt off so quickly that, by this season next year you will need a new wardrobe! I went from a size 22 to a size 8, sometimes a 6! You may not be able to imagine it today, but I promise you, if you eat healthy foods prepared in a healthy way, avoiding sweets and junk, especially alcohol, then you will change your body— permanently. You truly are what you eat. You have to want to do it!!

I gave up bread for Lent this past year. Talk about a sacrifice! Surprisingly, I have managed to stay away from it in a big way. Let me tell you, I have noticed a big change in my energy level! I am not tired after a meal now! As for the wine, I gave recently it up too! A glass of Merlot just doesn't taste as good, especially without the standard bread and butter accompaniment! Communion *was* always my favorite part of mass.

All this giving up of things I used to love has really opened up so much more life for me! **Sublimating potentially unhealthy desires allows for much more creative thought and energy!** I thought how hypocritical it would be if I went out for a few drinks and ate a huge meal while telling you that you shouldn't! After two (or three!) glasses of wine, I may have fuzzy recollections of parties and special moments before. Releasing myself from those habits (I *rarely* drink alcohol now), I see the world through new "rose-colored glasses"— everything so clear and fresh! I highly recommend beating all of your vices, one at a time. Rome wasn't built in a day, nor can you change 20+ years of habits and lifestyle overnight, but in a year you can!

Change is never easy, but it is possible, and much easier if you stick to the basic principles given you here. You have to want it. And you have to want to avoid the negative aspect of refusal to change. Something needs to get you going from behind, and pulling you forward in front— the carrot and the stick theory.

Creating a picture of a *"new life"*

To help yourself along the way, one thing you may wish to do is to make a wish poster. I used old pictures of myself when I was thin, and a few cut out pictures out of some familiar women's mags, along with pictures of beautiful clothes and some pretty jewelry. I would also find some pictures of settings and other beautiful backgrounds in which I imagined myself. It was a collage of looks, places, settings—a complete scene of the many things that motivated me. I placed my poster board where I would see it when I got up in the morning (near the bathroom mirror is an ideal place). Each morning, I looked at my "wish poster" and visualized myself not only thin, but healthy, happy, and full of life! You may know Mark Victor Hansen from the *Chicken Soup...* books. He will tell you that "visualization is realization," because anything must first happen in your mind before it can become a reality! So visualize each day the life you want to be living with every detail. In a matter of days, that picture will become more and more discernible, and soon, crystal clear!! You will be then making it a reality. *This really worked for me, especially since I never really accepted the look of "FAT Julia."* In doing this, it will help you **focus your sites on the future!**

With weight loss, I suggest you look around and evaluate the habits and behaviors of those you consider thin. Do they eat as you now do? Most likely they do not. Thin people tend to eat more slowly, serve themselves moderate portions and generally steer clear of the high in fat and fried foods. You don't often see people with great bodies at the fried chicken fast food spots! They do not look, nor act deprived. They enjoy food for food's sake, rather as nourishment NOT fulfillment or pleasure!

Each day, make the decision to live a healthy life and commit yourself to achieving it. Make it your goal, make it your dream. A wise man once told me, "make no small dreams for there is no magic in them." You need to see that living a full, healthy and complete life does have a certain amount of magic about it! Look at children, everything they do is FUN, so full of life, so in awe of it, so full of magic! Just because we are older doesn't mean we can't live our lives with those same elements of magic and awe present! Magic is so positive, so energizing! Life is an adventure and is meant to be lived that way! *What a boring existence to have your days revolve around what food to eat and what is on television!* Soon it will become second nature, ingrained in your thoughts. Remind yourself daily that achieving your goal will feel a lot better (for a lot longer) than the unhealthy food will taste. Going to the park with your kids, or hiking will provide you with memories that will last a lot longer than what happened on your favorite show! Make yourself believe that you are special, much more than a body with too much food in it!

There's nothing rigid about what you need to do here— no daily menus, or high cost payments per pound, no diets to follow— only simple guidelines. You decide what to eat, when and how much. I've advised you what not to eat and equipped you with my recipes and grocery list (and hopefully some of my boundless energy and renewed love of life!). I want to inspire you and jump-start you to take action! Ultimately, it is *your* decision to live each day to its fullest that will propel you toward your goals!

REWARDS

Throughout this book, I've assured you that this is not a rigid, restrictive diet plan, but rather a transition to a healthy, energetic way of life. That's not to say the transition is always easy. Along the way we all need some motivation to keep us going— some positive reinforcement when things get ho-hum. After 4 years of keeping my weight off certainly there are times that I would love to eat pastries, cakes, pies, pasta with cream sauce, etc. But I know that I want to continue living the fit, active and healthy life that I am now living!!

It is important to reward yourself when you **do** meet most of your goals. I came to crave my rewards more than I ever craved ice cream. I think that system is the key to how I have kept the weight off this long and will most likely never gain it back! I still treat myself to the pampering, self-indulgent and soothing rewards now that I did from day one of this, my last diet! There is nothing wrong with wanting to look and feel your best— and rewarding yourself for working to achieve it! I never went on something and therefore a day has not yet arrived that I need to go off of it. I treat myself well, and believe in holding highest of standards in everything. After all, aren't you worth it?

Rewards give you the daily encouragement needed to continue with being successful. The life you can lead from here on out *is* your goal. Becoming fit and healthy became a burning desire in my mind, because I realized that I wanted to *live*! I didn't want to have my heart give out before I was ready to quit living! I have two young children and I really want to watch them grow up! Raising kids is a huge task, filled with a lot of joy, you get one chance to do it right! And enjoying time with them was certainly a reward I didn't want to miss out on.

Taking Control of Life!

I haven't yet reached a day when I have wanted to say to myself, "Julia, aren't you tired of treating yourself so good and feeling so good about yourself. Let's go back to those self defeating behaviors!" I really can't see a day that I would ever feel that way! **Life today is itself a reward**. Taking each day as an opportunity to succeed with every action *is* a reward! Give thanks each day the Lord has made!

One thing I never did was weigh myself, although I could tell when I had lost a substantial amount of weight because my clothes would be bigger. When my clothes seemed a bit bigger, as a special treat I'd go to a movie or a museum, usually by myself just to get a break and focus on other great things. For example, after losing enough weight to fit in non-plus sized jeans again, I **treated myself to a full hour massage— heaven on earth!** The choices are endless— anything you enjoy (that is not food related of course) is a great way to reward yourself.

Although a new outfit is a special treat, I don't recommend purchasing a lot of new clothes along the way. Not only might this get you comfortable at a weight that is short of your goal, but you will also be wasting clothes once you've lost more weight to make them too big. Try purchasing accessories to revitalize an outfit or an item that will be easier to take in than a dress or suit. This is not to say you shouldn't buy a special outfit or a few new things, but don't do the new wardrobe bit until you have reached your goal!

One month after buying a size 12, I was a size 10 jean, and soon they were baggy, too. I wasted money not waiting a little bit longer! Amazed with my progress, I loved the fact that I was approaching my goal. I could wear nice business suits, jeans and shorts. I finally felt terrific in clothes again. My rewards gave me *motivation to continue each step of the way. I was beginning to feel like a woman again. I wasn't just a mom anymore or someone's discarded wife! It was great to **feel alive and vibrant**—for the first time in years!*

In order to have rewards, you need to know what you are rewarding yourself for. Establish small goals for yourself, both long and short term goals. Then create a of list things that you would want as a reward or treat once you meet that goal. For example, when I went two weeks with out eating ANY ice cream, then I went and had a full set of nails put on! What ever it is that will make you work hard to earn it! I have recommended to people that they buy tickets to a concert or event coming to town in a month or so; if you don't meet your goals set to achieve by then, you don't go! You have to give the tickets away! Not an easy thing to do, but living 20 years less because of an unhealthy body is no reason to celebrate!

You will learn to enjoy these treats so that nothing will get in your way! Think of the science experiment with Pavlov and his dogs. He could make them do anything just for their treats! You are an intelligent, rational individual, who can be motivated by positive rewards— just define 'em first!

Using a rewards system, you are setting yourself up for success! You are taking the control of your life back, not putting yourself on some diet that will only doom you to failure. It will work for you. Human beings are predictable creatures— we seek pleasure, that which makes us feel good. You will want to reach them again and again! I still use this system and I am still not dieting. Rewards are necessary in all we do! When I am done writing, responding to e-mails or with a day of telephone calls, I will spend time with the children, go somewhere on the weekend for the day, or just see a movie! I do it so I'm always looking forward to accomplishing a goal. Sometimes just moving on to the next task and getting excited about it, is rewarding enough!

Make each day a new life!

Taking each day as the first day of the rest of my life, I treat it as a completely separate and new beginning. So when I wake up, I am thinking of the ways I will work on my mental, physical, spiritual, and even financial health. If I am further than I was when I awoke, then I have improved. In this way I am following this adage:

"Live in the present, learn from the past, and plan for the future."

I don't want to be a 90 year old burden to my family, unhealthy and in need of a medic just to get out of a chair. I want everyday for the rest of my life to be full of quality. There is a lot left on this earth that I want to do! My long term goals include traveling the world, meeting people from all over the globe, and learning about the history of some of my favorite places. Then there are some short term goals— those weekly and monthly targets that I shoot for.

Make your goal sheet look something like this:

WEEK 1....... no _____ (ice cream was mine)
WEEK 2....... no _____ ("   ")

Reward: _____ (manicure was mine)

WEEK 3.......walk 20 minutes 3 times, no_____
WEEK 4.......walk 25 minutes 3 times, no_____

Reward: _____ (haircut/style for me)

WEEK 5........walk 30 minutes 4 times, no_____
WEE K 6.......walk 35 minutes 4 times, no_____
   Bake cookies for the local fire department

Reward: _____ (off to a museum)

3 month goal:_____ (reward here)
6 month goal:_____ ("   ")
1 year goal:_____ ("   ")

Review after each week, and update each month.

By the end of six weeks, you will most likely be at least 10 pounds thinner, you will definitely be looking better— new nails, and maybe with a new hairdo, and possibly some new knowledge from a museum! I guarantee that people will ask what you have done differently! You will most likely have more energy and be feeling proud of yourself for reaching your goals! When you have lost weight you find that it seemed so easy! You weren't counting calories, you weren't watching what food groups you were combining! You were simply eating healthy foods and drinking a lot of water. It is about that easy!

It is important that you identify what things will work for you as rewards. It is different for each person, if there are any men reading this book, you can tell it is definitely written from a female perspective! I am a woman, therefore I think like a woman, I don't know what type of stuff would motivate a guy, you have to do that for me! E-mail me and tell me what stuff moves men to action, I really would like to know, maybe give me some insight into the male psyche! Is it really new power tools or a work bench that does it for men? Would a massage even tempt you? Let me know, please! Maybe the motivation will be to meet some newly svelte woman who has been following my advise and is now thin and very positive about life!! That's a nice thought!

For women I can think many ways to reward yourself for healthy eating as you slim

Beauty care REWARDS

down, and through the years as you keep the weight off. Right now you may not like what you see when you look in the mirror. If so, you are focusing on the damage that having too much food in you is doing to your body. What do you see if you look past that? Pretty eyes, a nice smile, a good complexion? What about your hair, have you let it go as well as your body? While it may take time to get your body back to a normal weight, you can fix your hair right now! You can buy a new shade of lipstick today! Why not have a home make-up party or go to one of the make up counters at the mall and have them make you up! If you are like I was, you have forgotten what a beautiful woman lies beneath the layers of fat. Let her out! Let her start to show the world what you've been hiding! Even at 250 or more pounds, you are still beautiful, show it to the world!!

I would reach a short term goal before spending money on anything. But one month is not far away, so you can plan now. I recently saw a line of products I had never seen before— a Hollywood wife developed them and looked great, so I ordered some! You really don't have to leave your home to get great deals! The Internet and cable are really making our lives so easy— QVC is a great source! Don't fall into the trap of using this technology to get lazy though, use it to free up your time so that rather than running around the mall, you can be at the park, or at a step aerobics class! Something that is healthy and good for you!

Beauty reward items

Some reward items: eye shadows, lip sticks and liners, foundation, mascara, nail polish, and all the fun products for manicures and pedicures. (I have a stone buffer in my shower and love to rub my feet with it every couple of days—very pampering!), new shampoo, conditioner, body washes; try all the great aroma therapy that is out now; masks, exfoliant and more! The list really is endless!

Make-up is not the only thing that you can do along the lines of beautification. I utilized plenty of services, each one more indulgent and pampering than the next as I reached each new goal! Manicures, pedicures, and facials are a wonderful treat! You deserve to spend a little time and a little money on yourself! I promise you that doing this will make you feel so revived, like a new woman! If money is a concern, I would first see if there is a cosmetology school in your area. If so, usually you can get services performed by students at <u>very</u> reduced costs! There are also many products available at local drug stores that can allow you to do these treats on yourself, the end result is the same. Bright red nail polished fingers make it easier to pass up the french fries, you wouldn't want to mess up your pretty nails, would you?!

A new haircut, perm or color immediately changes your outward appearance! Personally, I would recommend letting your hair grow long. When I was obese, I wore my hair as short as a man's- and bit my nails! I have observed that many women are like I was. When we are overweight, I guess sub-consciously we don't think it matters. We think that we look so terrible that we tell ourselves 'what will make-up or a new hairdo change'! It is the attitude that changes with it! Look at Emme, a "plus size model", she is "overweight" and beautiful- I have seen her in person, she doesn't look "fat" to me! Maybe it is because she does put importance on how she looks, and always is made up and in nice clothing.

Decide today that you are worthwhile and deserve the best out of life! It starts with you! YOU have to look in the mirror, like what you see, change what you can improve, accept what you can't and learn to love yourself and treat yourself with respect. If you respected yourself, you would NOT eat a half gallon of ice cream at a time. NO WAY!

Massages and a body polishing are great treats! Sure, the thought of stranger seeing you practically naked is frightening. However after you have lost 25 or 50 pounds, you won't mind! It is their job, they have seen all different types of bodies and won't mind yours! They will rally around your weight loss and encourage you to keep going. Most people involved in this field are health conscious, many holistic. They realize what is on the inside needs nourishment and that massage provides a great stress relieving benefit!

Being at ease!

Buy some scented candles. Burning them a night gives such a nice peaceful scent around the house and creates the same mood. This will give you that fresh smell of vanilla or autumn floating throughout your home. A bouquet of fresh flowers on your kitchen or dining room table, will make you feel special, putting mother nature's goodness in the air (now that your eating the same, too!). Fresh flowers always boost my spirits, I never mind getting them for the house. How about buying a new CD that is a relaxing 'new age' sound? Eat healthy for a month and treat yourself to the music that you will be in heaven with! Great for listening to while you take a bath.

The key to this "rewards" system is to remember that you may only do these things if and only if you earn them! By that I mean, successfully meeting the goal that you placed on the particular reward. Make your goal a worthwhile and meaningful goal that you can be proud of, and your reward will be just the, uh, "icing on the cake?"... well, a great added bonus!

Change your surroundings

Creating a revitalizing and fresh atmosphere is essential to well-being! I really believe this! It sets the stage for all that you do. Think about it for a moment, if a stranger walked into your house today, right now, what would it say about you? Are there dishes strewn about in the kitchen, papers stacked on the floor, an overflowing trash bag waiting to be taken outside? Are the beds made, are the toys neatly arranged, is the furniture in need of replacing or at least slip covering, are there any plants around to supply fresh oxygen? I know that when I was overweight, it is safe to say that my home was in complete disarray! One extremely indulgent reward that I allow myself once in awhile is using a maid service! For $50 or so, you can have someone come and clean your house top to bottom! Working together, you can make your environment castle-like! You will feel like a queen! And a queen always take care of her home and health!

Anything that you do to reward yourself that enhances the quality of your surroundings will only further motivate you to keep going! Who wouldn't want their house looking showroom perfect! While you are fixing your body, you can be "getting your house in order," too! Successful, motivated, physically fit people do not live in squalor! By the time your weight is off, you will be accustomed to living graciously, and will expect the best for yourself.

Rewards don't have to cost money either. The following page lists some of mine. Begin to make one for you! Remember, it must come from within— something you desire and enjoy that will help you grow in every area of your health!

A list of possible rewards!

Grow your own flowers!   Plan a vacation
Start your own garden   Buy plants for home
Visit the local zoo   Buy a new CD
Take a trip to a museum   Burn a scented candle
Take a walk in a park   Get you hair done
Go on a scenic bike ride   Get your nails done
Take a country walk   Paint a room
Take a city walk   Get new clothes

Listen to relaxing music
Go to a movie
Read an interesting book
Study a new subject
Contribute time to a charity
Volunteer at a local school
Do a painting
Learn the use of a computer
Take up a sport (a great idea!)
Sew a new outfit

New curtains
Flowers
A massage
Get a pet
take up a 2nd language
visit a historic place
Go to the library
Teach a child to read
—tennis, swimming,
take up woodworking

EXTRAVAGANT REWARDS

Buy a new car
Get cosmetic surgery
New jewelry

Go to Paris
Travel to Egypt
A new house

One mention about the few things here. I mentioned it before, the reason we don't live up to our full potential is because we don't dream big enough. Our dreams and rewards need to be big enough to get us excited each day! Make the most exciting thing you could ever do in your lifetime stand out on your list. That will spur you into action!

Mental exercise

There are few better treats that one can give themselves than a new book, or rereading an old favorite! Without sounding like a preacher, I would even recommend the Bible. I am trying to read it front to back. It a fascinating Book with everything on living well. Any book that contains information on interesting facts or anything of interest to you is an excellent way to develop your mind. Many people with higher degrees lose their mental sharpness because they no longer study. Although real life experiences can not be substituted with reading, learning about a subject that requires reading is a great mental exercise that can move your focus to the amazing things that actually exist in this universe of ours...or possibly of someone else's, too!

Moving ahead for a moment, I'd like to discuss the future— your future. Although it may seem premature, I'd

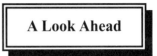

A Look Ahead

like to help prepare you for what lies ahead. As I achieved success through my program, I wasn't always prepared for the emotional and psychological changes that accompany a significant weight loss, but I want you to be, or at least anticipate some.

Life is different as a thin person. If you're currently in a relationship, it's likely to change— hopefully, for the better if your partner is supportive and sensitive. You may notice that many of the people in your life were very comfortable with and accustomed to you being overweight. You've seen the news stories about someone wearing a "fat suit," venturing out to seek employment only to be treated with inferiority. The woman wearing the fat suit takes her impressive resume in to a business and applies for a job, she is told that she isn't qualified or that the job has been filled. Next, "Betty Bombshell" walks in and the employer fawns all over her, asking when she can start, despite the fact the previous prospect was much more qualified for the job! Even if you are not aware of it, you yourself have been treated less than fairly at some time or another. I know that while heavy I was paid much less than women whom I out-produced! This I have physical proof of! Of course, back then, the fat, depressed woman I was, didn't have the ability to take action. ***No one ever said life is fair, but you can literally tip the scales in your favor now, if you want to!*** You can unzip and remove that fat suit. As you step out, be prepared to face a brave new world!

Appearing different

People now treat me with more respect than when I was fat. Perhaps it's because I see myself differently now that I am slim and feel that I look good. When I saw myself "fat" and minimized my self-worth, people treated me the way I felt I deserved to be treated. It's time to stop the circle of self-defeating thoughts and behaviors. It's not easy to be confident when you are obese and angry with yourself. No matter how much weight you loose, you are the same person, just shining with more life and enthusiasm. You will have a renewed sense of self, but essentially, you will be the same. The world will think that you are somehow a different person. It is the opposite of how they see you today. The world views us as lazy if we are overweight. I'm sure you are far from lazy. You just aren't using your efforts in the most constructive way to lose weight!

As you begin to slim down, wait for the looks you will get from strangers! These are the same ones who, when you were overweight, stared and glared when you ordered a Mrs. Field's™ cookie. They made you feel as if you were committing a crime and should be ashamed for ordering anything "fattening." Now that I'm thin, I sometimes wonder what the looks are for now!

I think that respect is necessary for those who have too much food in them as well as for those who do not. One of my readers has lost 65 lbs. so far, and while at a recent family reunion she said her relatives stopped just shy of actually saying how fat she used to be! In their own way, I am sure they meant no insult, but this could be very unpleasant! They should have commented on how great and healthy she looked now, not dwell on the past! She claimed the Aunties were offering her pie repeatedly telling her she didn't want to get too thin! She still had 50 pounds that she wanted to lose! She was glad to see her aunts, but shouldn't have to eat their pies to show that she loves them!

As you transform yourself to the svelte swan, the difference is amazing and, fortunately, it is a gradual change. You won't wake up tomorrow morning and suddenly be THIN. However, by the time you are, your mind set will be almost there, too, if you follow my self-esteem building regime. I still find myself looking in the mirror (perhaps a little too much), amazed that the reflection I see is really me!

If you had a crystal ball and could look into the future, you would see that I am right. A year from now, your life will be different than it is today. Better, healthier and more active... It is impossible *not* to change if you lose a 100 pounds! I figure I could carry a small gymnast around all day on my back and still not match the stress that I was putting on my heart when I was 130 lbs heavier! Think about that— could you pick up a 100 lb. sack of flour, or a 100 lb. weight in the gym? I carried that much and more around everyday for 8 years of my life! I couldn't carry 100 lbs. around now if I wanted to! Little wonder getting out of a movie theater seat was such a chore, or lifting myself up out of the bathtub— I practically needed a crane to get up when I was 9 months pregnant with Clark! Not only was I obese, I had a baby filling up my body as well (and overflowing the tub!) That was then.

Setting goals for yourself is fundamental! We often set up reward systems for our children.. 'make your bed, get a dollar', etc. for ourselves we expect that we will do the things that we want or need to do, without rewards. You might, however, you are much more likely to do the things you need to do if there is a reward at the other end waiting for you! We are all Pavlov's dogs, so to speak!

After I had lost my weight, I didn't quit setting goals for myself. Life should always be about growing and changing, looking for new challenges, if it's not, that's when we get into trouble, boredom!! When do you eat?....when you are bored!! Reaching your goals provides you with such a sense of accomplishment, often times, that in itself is a great reward! After I had lost 130 pounds, I thought about what I wanted out of life, what was next for me, I wrote down a list of goals, or things that I wanted to do.

1. Write my story, a book.
2. Help other women better their lives.
3. Become Mrs. Missouri—a beauty queen!?
4. Have another baby.
5. Be happy forever.
6. Own a successful business.
7. Attend the Oscars ceremony.

When I wrote this list, a lot of things on it seemed too far fetched or impossible to me, but none the less, they represent things that I would really like to do. As of this day, I have fulfilled 5 out of the 7! When I was a little girl, I watched Miss USA and dreamed that one day I would do that. I never did, I got married young and became obese instead. Well guess what, this coming July, I will be representing my state as Mrs. Missouri in the Mrs. United States of America contest! That might not be what everyone aspires to do, but for a woman who weighed 270 lbs., it is a dream come true! Once you write something down, make it real and then begin working to make it happen you unleash untapped power—watch out world! Nothing but **YOU** can stop you from reaching your goals! In the same respect, no one except for **YOU** can fulfill them either!

Taking Control of Life!

PART

III

"The Second Chapter"

"The Second Chapter"

I have shared a lot of my life with you, this probably reads more like a cheesy novel than a diet book (do we see that Demi-Moore-starring movie in the future?! Tell Mr. Spielberg we can talk!). You are perhaps wondering what happened to me after I threw my husband out. A lot! I continued to eat sensibly, went to counseling and became a better mother. I threw myself into my job. I had to be productive now, and the option of poverty scared me too much. I had seen the statistics of women who get divorced—losing their homes, living on one income and some child support, no room for any life's extras. I made ends meet— barely! My parents got very involved in my life. I didn't make it easy on them to help, but help they did! I could always count on them to buy the winter coats for the kids or get a good meal if we needed it! I was lucky. Little actually changed for us. I got to keep the house, although with all the debt. He left with little, but none of the debt either. (I am *still* paying off his truck.) But, I got the kids! All the money in the world couldn't buy the joy they give to my life!

Those first few months alone were scary. Even though my ex had rarely been at home, I never felt as alone as I did when I knew he was never coming back home. I shed a lot of tears in those all too quite late hours! I even had the kids sleep in bed with me, I just couldn't stand that I had no one to hold or to hold me. Even though I hadn't really had it for so long by then, the thought of knowing that there was no chance I would was an empty feeling that I can't express. I would have to leave writing that eloquent to the Danielle Steele or Hemingways of the world. I am just a normal woman. But it hurt, I ached inside. I felt so inadequate! What did this woman have that I didn't! What was wrong with me! I pulled the kids close to me and slept, comforted in the fact that I was at least 'good enough' for them to love me!

Taking Control of Life!

Fall approached quickly, my favorite time of the year! I was purposely wearing tight blue jeans again, the first time in 8 years! I felt so energized on those fall mornings to pull blue jeans on and a cute shirt, I was actually beginning to look like all the non-obese moms dropping their kids at school, although they would be returning home to their happy marriages in their minivans! I was jealous! I wanted the perfect suburban life that I was surrounded by! I wanted the loving husband and secure family life!

SPOOKY!!

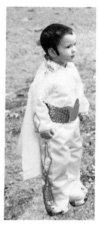

The kids and I had a great Halloween that year, our first holiday alone. Taylor was the scariest looking witch you have ever seen. Clark wouldn't go near her and kept crying for his *"real"* 'sissy'! I dressed Clark up as 'Tiny Elvis.' I spray painted his hair black, painted on sideburns and had the gold lame jumpsuit to complete the look! It was a great day! We laughed, giggled and didn't feel like anything was missing, the day was complete!

I can't help but remember one Halloween a few years ago, I had dressed Taylor as a bride, she even wore my veil! I sewed pearl and sequins on her dress, adding lace and appliques. She was stunning, even if she was only 5! Clark was a new born, I put him in the cutest baby Tuxedo pj outfit! Red bow tie and all! They were so adorable! 'Frog baby' looked like "Uncle Fester" then! (Nicknamed such by my sister and her husband, they couldn't quit laughing when they saw the pictures, Uncle Fester!...... they nearly cried they laughed so hard!) I took the kids everywhere that afternoon and evening, showing them off and trick or treating to all the homes of our family and friends. What a fun day that had been, but sadly, something, or someone as it were, was missed and wanted! He was busy, it was hunting season and "Halloween was for kids" he exclaimed as he left for the weekend.

What a difference a few years makes! I can honestly say I didn't think about what was wrong, but all of the good things that were right. The fact that I was on my own with the kids allowed me to realize all of these good things, and enjoy life, and grow each day.

The children now started going over to their dads on the nights he had them. I, for the first time in years, had some free time, time that I could focus on doing self-building activities. It allowed me some freedom. It wasn't such a bad thing.

At first I felt totally lost. With the children gone I had absolutely nothing to do, they had been my life for years. I couldn't figure out what I should do, I had seen all the latest movies— alone, and the house was spotless. One of my best girlfriends was also single so we started going out to have fun together. She allowed me to tag along with her work buddies to happy hours. What a difference 10 years makes!! The singles scene was a lot different now than I remembered it! I never had trouble meeting guys before, I had my pick and choose. Now, I was slightly chunky, middle aged and had two kids. Just what your average good-looking bachelor is looking for!

The dating scene...again?

My confidence *was* coming back, along with

my waist line. I decided to take control of my life in a bold manner, I entered the 90's! Even at the risk of unmerciful teasing by my girlfriends, I took out an ad in the personals section of the local paper. I have to tell you, those things are "weirdo" magnets! It was great to be able to say that I had a date, but too many questions to answer as to where we met, how long had I known him, etc... My family and friends were more concerned with my love life than they were when I was 18! Some of my dates were a lot of fun, most of them were in the same boat as I was— divorced and trying to restart their lives. I felt sorry for most of them. They were middle aged guys, missing their kids, losing their hair, not a lot of money to date with after paying child support. I felt sorry for me, was this what life was going to be like? The few that acted like they liked me, were looking for a place to live and someone to support them. I was much more in the need of someone to do all that for me!

I found a few men who were great company, successful and they became my regular date night guys. Nice dinners out and an occasional kiss. I was actually getting comfortable with my new life. At least I was going out and finding that others were interested in me. My dad thought that I was dating too soon, especially given that my divorce wasn't final yet. I figured that since my husband had been dating the same woman for 3 years now, the courts wouldn't fault me too much for dating occasionally!

I had even begun to make friends with some of my coworkers and started going out to happy hour and such with them. Before, I always had to rush home to get the kids, now their dad actually was doing his fair share. They were getting to know their dad, and I was developing a bit of a social life once again. One guy I worked with kept swearing that he and I were meant to be together and he kept asking me out. I was crazy about him as a friend, he made me laugh and we had a great time with each other, but he just didn't interest me as a boyfriend or role model for my kids. Dating is a lot more complicated when you have to consider, ...what if this worked out, how would he be with the kids...? I ended up screening many guys off the list earlier than I would have without kids, many of them would have made the cut years ago. I had to consider my actions much, more seriously than 15 years ago, it wasn't just me that my decisions affected! If my children didn't warm to someone the first time they met him, he was off the team. Kids are great judges of character, I wasn't obviously, so I let them guide me through this time!

Let's jump ahead a few months— I was now a 115 pounds thinner. I looked and felt like a new woman. I must, even the ex tried to get me interested in fooling around with him! He was at the house moving some furniture around for me and actually had the nerve to hit on me! I didn't even consider that as an option for one second. Oh well, I was reading a lot of great books at night. That kept my mind on other creative things. Besides, after losing 115 pounds, I looked a lot better in clothes, but out of them, I was resembling a Shar-Pei puppy, only not as cute! I hoped that someday I would be lucky enough to fall in love again and could actually be naked in front of a man other than my doctor— that thought terrified me!!

A surgical solution?

Because I had so much noticeable damage to my skin from being overweight, I sought an opinion from a cosmetic surgeon to see what my options were. After many consultations and many opinions from different physicians, I felt I had met with one of the best. I only wanted a couple of things corrected, and believed that

I would feel better about myself. I actually considered it somewhat of a reward for my weight loss accomplishment. My family did not agree with my decision to have surgery, they encouraged me to work out and let nature takes it's course. Every doctor I consulted with had convinced me that it would be very difficult to return my sagging body to it's pre-obese state. (Although, a few mentioned that exercise <u>during</u> my weight loss would have increased the chances). Nothing would shrink my skin, stretched beyond imagination from years of too much food in it, back to normal. Nothing except a nip here and a tuck there. I was sold. One draw back, the surgeon said that if I intended on staying thin, I would need to incorporate regular exercise into my life. "What? I just lost 100 pounds, I don't need exercise." I walked with the kids around the park, and figured that was enough. I believed that I was in fact the queen of weight loss at this point in my life, who was he to tell me differently? I really wasn't a fan of exercising. Given my 90's lifestyle, I decided to give a personal trainer a try. Think about this picture: Julia, 100 pounds thinner, divorced, dating again, having fun again, giving myself great rewards to boost my self- esteem, contemplating cosmetic surgery and now a trainer! I was almost Ivana Trump! Look at me go! I eventually did have my surgery, a nip and tuck to correct *some* of the damage, but not for taking off any weight.

Things were moving along just fine, we had our first Christmas alone. My ex must have been missing his family, he asked if he could spend the night and watch the kids wake up to see Santa's presents under the tree. He was usually out with his best friend or already asleep by then. I obliged, thinking of the children. (Of course, he slept on the couch.) I would arrange all the presents under the tree, drink my no longer warm milk and cookies, and make reindeer tracks outside in the snow! I would move ashes around in the fireplace to make it look like Santa fell down! The next day was nice for the kids. It's hard not to be in the spirit of the holidays on Christmas.

New Year's Eve rolled around, and I let the kids have a sip of champaign before they went to bed. I drank the whole bottle— not too healthy, and not too smart.

A new year, a new me. I was really beginning to like being on my own. I didn't have time to sulk anymore. I only focused on what needed to be done. Things were moving along well. I was doing great at my job— the top producer! My boss was actually paying me more now, too. I often wonder about the timing. When I was heavy and asked for a raise, I never got one. Now I strutted into his office looking better and got exactly what I asked for. It was good knowing and feeling confident, the results being a by-product of my achievement.

I was seeing one guy more than the rest, my friends at work called him "the bowler." Funny thing is that he didn't bowl that I knew of. He was very conservative, in a Republican sort of way. I was playing it safe, I was going for an older secure man. In a way, I wanted to be pampered a little. I had asked him to escort me to an office holiday party. I was teased for weeks! Maybe I was beginning to see their point. I was rather full of life for someone nearing the end of theirs— or closer, anyway. But it beat sitting home alone on a Saturday night and it sure beat a bar scene.

A new guy!!... Oh, my!

I have told you life has a way of sneaking up on us and to be careful out there. Little did I heed my own advice! My fat-free lunch group at work was a huge success. We became very cliquey, not just anyone could be part of it now. You had to be committed to healthy eating and making good tasting dishes, and it had become as much a social event as a meal!

A new guy had began working in our office, a doctor of all things. What he was doing there was a mystery to me. He was young, very young (at least by all appearances), and well groomed. What did he want to hang out with us eccentric recruiters for? "We recruit doctors to go to work for various hospitals and HMOs, we don't hire them to work with us," I thought. He indeed seemed out of place. The guys in my office smoked too much, drank on their off hours and complained about everything. This guy was very positive and up beat.   And did I mention handsome, very handsome! — and young, he looked 18!

He wormed his way into my lunch club— to eat! He hadn't yet brought his "contributory" meal. The day came that the young doctor Pat finally brought his lunch offering for the group.   I insisted that he must have made mommy stay up all night and cook for him. It was *way* to good to be low fat and certainly not made by his well manicured hands! Pasta shells stuffed with spinach, and it was delicious— I was impressed by the young-looking Dr.'s skill. *Can you detect that I hazed him a bit?* One day he informed me rather heatedly of his age, and that I could cease and desist with the teasing at anytime! Well, the young Dr. Pat was feisty, too!

Our boss had paired him with a different worker in my office to learn the business. Now wouldn't you put your bright young star with the best producer in the company? Not where I worked, that would have been a positive way to run the company. They were much more into the slaves-in-the- galley method of management. My boss would actually parade through the office shouting, "on the phone or on the bus!" One day Pat asked to work with me, he said he liked my energy and style. His request was of course denied, as even though I was the top producer, I had the worst work ethic known to corporate America! I was always 20 minutes late everyday and left by 2:30 or 3:00 most days. As a business owner, you really didn't want me influencing your workers, I was dismissed as a freak of nature, an oddity! Dr. Pat began to ask my opinion on deals he had working and we struck up a friendship. He was super intelligent (a mensa the guys claimed), very funny, healthy and I enjoyed his companionship! This went on for about 3 weeks. Eventually we were working together, as I don't think the boss could really say much about it, considering we were doing well.

THE magical kiss

One Friday afternoon, where all the employees of the company were meeting, "the bowler" met me there to take me out to dinner. My co-workers were making their comments about him from afar. Dr. Pat took one look at him and declared that he wasn't for me. I asked "do tell, who is for me "young" Dr. Pat?!" He replied— "I don't know, maybe someone more like me?" — but not this 'bowler!' On my way out, Dr. Pat proceeded to give me a "good-evening" kiss good-bye. He kissed my neck. The right side of my neck was on fire and it spread through the entire right side of my body!!! Wow! They should bottle that boy up and sell him, I thought! Needless to say, my date with "the bowler" was not as exciting! My mind was on my neck all night!-talk about a pain in the neck! The young Dr. Pat was becoming one!

The next night, everyone from my office came over to my house to cocktail and then go to a movie, Mr. Holland's Opus. Everyone was there, and we were all laughing and having fun. As I look towards my entry foyer I see in my front door walking the "young" and extremely good looking Dr. Pat. He had on black cowboy boots, jeans, a black sweater, a black cashmere overcoat— *and a drop dead smile!!* I was a "goner!" "Shoot me now and put me out of my misery," I thought, as I stood there in *my* black cowboy boots, jeans, black velour turtleneck sweater, grabbing for my black wool coat. We were bookends, two peas in a pod, yin and yang, Lucy and Ricky, you name it, it would fit! He captured my heart as well as my attention for the rest of the evening! Needless to say, I didn't catch much of Mr. H's Opus— *heard it was good*!?

After a couple weeks of getting to know each other, and some informal dates, as we did work together, he asked me out on a real date. I gladly accepted. Accustomed as I was to dating now, I didn't put a lot of thought into what to wear. He, however, insisted that I wear black. OK, perhaps he was a bit demanding, but I obliged. When he arrived, I hadn't even gotten out of the bath, the kids kept him entertained as the babysitter told me that he (the "10" as the sitters nicknamed him!) must be in a hurry because he kept looking at his watch.

The date was something out of an old movie. He took me to a great German restaurant in town, we ate German food and drank German wine. He looked at his watch once or twice— I thought I was boring him! He asked for the check and said we would have to leave now. Oh well, at least I got to know him a little better, and we had a nice dinner. We could be good friends. As he pulled out of the parking lot, he turned the opposite direction from my house. Hmm...Where were we going? We ended up outside of the concert hall, the symphony concert hall! He had gotten tickets for us to hear the music of a German composer! I had dreamed of a date like this— a handsome man, dining, romance, the symphony— now I was living my dream. After the concert, my first, he again was doing the 'looking at his watch' bit. Darn, I knew it was too perfect, figuring the night was soon over. We rushed to a quiet little bar across town, he walked right up to a woman at a table and gave her a kiss on the cheek, then shook the hand of the man that she was with. His sister and her husband, and their company was just as enjoyable. A perfect date, one I had been waiting for 30+ years!

Leaving my office

The young doctor Pat quit his job soon thereafter to start his own consulting business. The sly dog, he had been in there merely to learn the ropes before going it alone. We didn't think our romance could remain secret for long and the gossip mongers were already licking their chops. They knew something was up by my smiling all the time and flowers delivered to me. I will cut to the chase so as to not bore you or share details that are my happy and wonderful memories best left in my heart where they belong!

Pat and I eloped to Las Vegas 6 months after our first date. Actually we are still on our first date since we have yet to spend any time apart from each other. It has been the happiest 3 years of my life. I have finally found a home! He loves me, he encourages my every idea and whim. He allows me the freedom to be myself and never ridicules me for my eccentric nature. He jumped right into fatherhood and has done it with grace, style and love. I could go on and on about his attributes but I will keep that to myself. *I wouldn't want to give the adulterous women of the world a new target, would I?!*

I will share one story of our life together with you to illustrate for you what a 'great husband' I have now! My darling little Taylor was in the hospital after breaking her arm at a playground in a local fast food chain (the type I never take them to anymore).

Pat was home caring for Clark, who had thrown up all over the car only hours earlier. I called him and I told him the situation, and being that he is a chiropractic physician (*he knows bones!*)— he gave me some comforting words. After speaking with the doctor, he assured me that she would be fine. I had to make all these decisions, allow them to operate on my baby, slice her open, put a pin in, scar her for life, general anesthesia.... The orthopedic surgeon said they had to perform the surgery immediately. I had no choice, she would lose the use of her arm if we waited any longer. Poor Taylor, she was scared and so upset. Her biggest concern was getting back to the slumber party she had been at! I kissed my beautiful little angel as they wheeled her away from me. I cried and prayed. Before long my dad was there by my side.

God bless my dad, he has always been there for me, no matter what! No matter how old I am, a hug from my dad eases my pain, but this time it only lessened it. This was my child in an operating room. Dad assured me she would be OK. I asked him: "what about the scar?" He said, "No one ever looks at Miss America's forearm!" His perspective on life brought a smile to my face. I waited nervously for 5 hours, then the doctor said she did great and would be fine.

I went home after 4 days at the hospital with nearly no time away— to sleep and take a shower. As I walked towards the house, I smelled cooking from inside. What a nice surprise! Patrick had cooked all afternoon, making me a beautiful dinner, with a bottle of chilled French wine open and poured for me. Soft jazz music was playing on the CD, the table was set with the fine china and flowers on the table. We ate in a peaceful, quite ambience, and after dinner he massaged me for an hour till I was sound asleep. I awoke a new woman, ready to face the results of surgery, knowing that I was truly loved, giving me the strength not to let my daughter see the fear in my eyes!

I was happy and felt that those around me were giving me great support in dealing with my daughter's trauma. I think it's true that *"the Lord helps those who help themselves."*

PART

IV

Managing a Healthy Life...

FOREVER!

In this last section, I have tried to condense all of the important points to living a successful life—health of mind, body, and soul! Follow these guidelines on a daily basis!

Weight-Management Musts

* Stay off the scale. The primary role of exercise is to burn calories but, at the same time, you are reshaping your body with muscle tissue that weighs more than fat tissue. Use your measurements, the way your clothes fit (even a body-fat analysis) as ways to evaluate your progress as well as your maintenance! Remember, you're not on a diet!

* Exercise your cardiovascular system three to five days each week for 20 to then 40 minutes using activities like walking, biking, stair climbing, cross-country skiing, swimming or circuit training with weights. To increase fat loss, build up to 60 minutes a day at a moderate pace. The "talk test" is a good indicator of intensity. It requires that you work out at a level that still allows you to talk or carry on a conversation comfortably during your activity. If you can't talk, you're not working out effectively!

* Include strength training two to three days a week in your exercise routine to shape muscles and build lean body mass. Muscle tissue raises your metabolism, making it easier to maintain your new weight. The craze in weight loss these days is muscle mass— the more you have it, the better your body burns calories! I recently read an article that says anaerobic exercise (strength training with weights) burns 500% more calories than aerobic exercise. Do it now!

* "Use it or lose it." Muscle tissue does not turn to fat once you stop training, but your body needs to be active. Although I don't know why or when you will "stop" training! You don't want to gain the fat back, do you? Muscle and fat cells are different substances in the body. Muscles shrink or atrophy without use so, this saying holds true as it should. The body requires maintenance just like your car. The big difference, of course, is that you can abuse your car and trade it in for a new one— unlike the body!

* **Establish a workout schedule** and stick to it, making it a habit. Find the time of day that best fits your schedule. If there is no available time in your schedule, you need to rearrange your priorities. Exercise IS a MUST component of your new habits and lifestyle. Scheduling workout times on your calendar can help you to squeeze exercise into your busy day. You can seek the help of a personal trainer just to help you establish a routine and a commitment to stick with it.

* **Set a long-term, six month goal for yourself**. Then, break that down into short term, weekly goals. For example, a long term goal could be dropping two sizes in your jeans. Your short term goal may be to walk (or treadmill) three miles by the second week (not stopping until you reach that point), and cross training with weights three days a week. By the way, if you are exercising at home and walking, use your car to measure the distance in order for you to get the correct mileage (be sure its a round trip!).

* **Set realistic goals.** A trainer can help establish a healthy weight for you based upon your height, frame size, age and body composition. With most everything you can set your own goals and reach them if you put your mind to it. But as for the body, weight loss at an accelerated pace is not only not healthy, it could be dangerous. Your body will be good to you if you are good to it. Fill out your goal sheet and stick to it!

* **Reward yourself** for small accomplishments along the way. Remember, I used the manicure, massage, and many others at the salon and spa. The many fabulous services at a spa and salon are a great way of rewarding herself for reaching goals.

* **Have fun** with your exercise. This is NOT a prison sentence! Realistically, you need to include exercise in your lifestyle forever, so, have some fun with it. Try new activities, take a class, listen to fun music, share your time with a buddy, or, as I did, see how much you can make your trainer laugh during the workout to keep her or him entertained!

* **Live a healthy lifestyle**—managing your weight is best accomplished through changes in lifestyle, habits and attitude— the foundation of getting on the road to health. The foundation of your new lifestyle involves things that are fun, alive, energetic, and inspiring. You will throw out some of the old habits and replace them with things you may never have considered. It can be a bit overwhelming at times, so it helps to surround yourself with a network of people who can support you, coach you, and motivate you to be your best. Most importantly, these people are positive and focused and getting the most out of life, which you want for yours too!

Discipline yourself by following these guidelines, and you will excel!

I thought it would be appropriate to include a typical day for me now (the basics), that keeps me healthy and fit, so you have at least a model of exactly what to do. Although most of what I describe it common sense, having an example to compare to is the easiest way to know if what you are doing is good or could be better. On the following page is an example of my typical day.

Monday / Wednesday / Friday
7:00 am up,, dress for aerobics, breakfast for kids
8:30 am kids to school and off to aerobics
9:45 am shower, dress, lite breakfast
10:30—3:30 work, job related duties
3:30 lite snack/lunch, veggies or salad
4:00 pick up kids from school
5:00 prepare dinner
6:00 pm lite dinner
7-8 pm spend time with the kids, their homework,
    bathing, etc.
8-9 pm return phone calls, e-mails, and letters
9:30 battle plan the next day's activities/ actions
read 30 minutes

Tuesday and Thursday
same schedule except 4:30 weight training instead of
8:30 aerobics, and earlier work hours

Saturday
9:00 am weight training and 30 minutes treadmill
morning tasks; afternoon with the kids, evening with
spouse

With a schedule that involves working 9-5 that doesn't
allow you to get away for exercise, and early morning aerobics
class or an early evening one will be a great benefit. Also it is
important to work in weight training into your exercise program
as building muscle tone will burn calories faster than you can ever
imagine! If you feel time a problem, remember, this is a lifestyle,
not a temporary schedule. In other words, you don't have time
not to! Just go for it!

Common Traits of Successful People

The following items are those that have been found to be present in the lives of people who are living fulfilling, successful, healthy lives. Having me give you my story and what I do will hopefully give you something to relate to—my struggle and the ability to overcome obstacles. Yet I understand everyone may have a different set of circumstances with which they are faced. In thinking about what could best serve you the reader, I concluded that if you knew what people who were considered successful in all areas of their lives were doing, then some general guidelines could be followed. I learned something myself when investigating the things that seemed to be present, because I also am always trying to keep growing and learning. One thing a wise man once told me that rings true: **"the more you know, the more you learn there is so much you don't know."**

Everyone may have their own definition of success, and living a fulfilling life. But how success was defined was very simple—focusing on the basic "dynamics" of life—that is, a healthy mind, body, soul, as well as financial security. This doesn't mean filthy rich or wealthy, just peace of mind when it comes to having a home, food, and other basic needs. Its important to have balance in your life. You would hate to be well off financially if you weren't in good health, and vice versa. You don't want to get to a point where one aspect of your life is successful while the other two or three or lacking. Growing in every area will prove more stable and longer lasting. Try following, or fulfilling, the points on the following pages, and watch your life grow!

Successful people have been found to:

1. Have a strong sense of purpose with their life!

Knowing what it is that your working toward, contributing to society, and carrying out with conviction, will keep your passion and enthusiasm for life alive and kicking!

Example: My purpose is helping others achieve their weight loss goals. This means that upon awakening each day I know that my actions are ultimately directed toward helping others (you!)with the tools, knowledge, and motivation to move toward a better life!— My purpose can change, but ultimately it is very rewarding to know the underlying theme always includes others!

2. Be motivated by a deep, personal set of beliefs.

By believing that you can make the world a better place, be it in one community, or the entire state, because deep down you know you can see things that need change for the better, you will move yourself to action. This results from your beliefs about people, about intentions, and any belief you have that is influencing your thoughts and actions today. Sitting around and complaining about the way things are or should be is taking a passive role. Getting out and doing something about it because of your beliefs is active!

3. Have a strong belief in God or a Supreme Being.

This is another consistency with happy and successful people. Practicing some form of religion has many benefits, most of which are probably known to you. Believing in God keeps us humble and reflective on our actions, behavior, and personal development. Remember, you are either growing or you are moving in the other direction— life is not stagnant.

Successful people have been found to:

4. Have written and well defined goals.

If you don't know where your going, how do you know when you get there? It has been said that most people spend more time planning a vacation than planning their lives. Write down your goals, even if it is just a six month goal. And with weekly goals as well, you will know when you get there! Write down each detail of your goals— especially WHY!

5. Have no fear of death.

Because of the inner strength derived from other points on this list, successful people realize that their time here is only temporary, and know the day will come for a new life. With this mind-set and stability, won't you be taking more chances in your life? Live strong, and live well.

6. Be in a loving relationship, usually married.

As you heard in my story, not having my husband anymore left me feeling empty. Although love must begin with yourself, the amount of energy, life, and happiness gained from giving and receiving love in a relationship is exponential! Two kindred souls are more powerful and stable together.

7. Eat healthy and exercise regularly.

I don't have to elaborate on this one, as you know the benefits of both. Providing the right nutrition and exercise gives your body, among many other things, one very important item— fresh oxygen. Plenty of water, fruits, vegetables, and exercise gives your body oxygen— a life sustaining (and thriving!) must!

8.   Sleep 6-8 hours per day.
Adequate rest is vital to replenishing our energy, and nourishing our mind and soul! Replenishing the body allow for more energy and passion for life!

Further Points for
Continued Positive Growth!!

> ## Make the decision each day to be the
> ## person you want to be!

Choose to be happy and you will be happy. If you think you can or can't do something, you'll be right! You decide what you want and are willing to accept for yourself. If you refuse to accept mediocrity in your life, there will be none.

It may sound philosophical but it's true. Ultimately, you make the decisions that will affect your life. You can choose to begin pursuing a better life right now, or you can opt to stay where you are. If you feel your life is fine the way it is, you're not going to grow. Even the most successful people need bigger and greater goals to keep them growing. So empower yourself, go out and grab it with all the gusto you can.

> ## Make the choice each day to live
> ## healthy-mentally, physically, spiritually!

Every day you must make the commitment to put only healthy things into your body. As I changed the food I put into my body, I even quit smoking, too! How can someone eat healthy, work out and then suck tar into their lungs? It's illogical!

Mentally, you must quit beating up on yourself. Be proud of who you are, the person inside. Feel confident of who you are because you are making every decision with mental clarity, and know that it is the right decision with all you do!

Spiritually, let those in your life know how you feel about them; be kind and friendly to the people that you encounter in your daily life. For every act of kindness that you do, it comes back tenfold to you—even if it just means more smiles in the world around you. Keep one on your face—you'll find it's contagious. I believe it all ties together. God teaches us to be kind to others and also to regard our bodies as temples. Taking care of each area of your life gives balance and makes progress easier.

Make fruits and vegetables your foods of choice

Believe it or not, I now crave kiwi the way I used to crave ice cream. Kiwi, can you imagine? It's true! I believe God created our bodies with fruit and vegetable consumption in mind. Our hands and arms are ideal for picking fruits from the trees.

I've discovered vegetables are wonderful, too. Try eating an entire red pepper, it's crispy and better than potato chips any day! No oil and salt to hold water and fat in your body like a potato chip does...YUCK!

Make fats and unhealthy foods your greatest enemies!

This, I believe, is the cornerstone of my healthy eating, and was the cornerstone of my weight loss. The number one worst enemy has to be the food source that made me overweight, unhealthy and unhappy. It has to be yours, too. If you had a friend who kept getting you in trouble, wouldn't you eventually quit associating with this person? If you didn't, your choice would be self-destructive and unwise. The time has to come for you to stop associating with fats and unhealthy foods. Make them your enemies.

> **Set a weekly goal for achievement!**

Your goal does not have to be to lose a given number of pounds each week. Remember, I didn't weigh myself in the beginning of my weight loss. Your goal could be to go seven days without eating a cookie, chips, or ice cream. Whatever the enemy, aiming to eliminate it completely, starting with a week at a time, can be a great goal!

If eating fruits and vegetables doesn't come easy to you, your goal could be to add two or three of each to your daily choices that week. That would be great!

Your goals must be set by you, with the willingness to sacrifice to meet them or they won't be meaningful. An unreasonable goal is ridiculous and meaningless. Set realistic goals, but make them goals you want desperately to achieve. Then when you achieve your goals, they'll provide you with the satisfaction and desire to keep going!

Look to where you're going, not where you've been!

Don't berate and beat yourself up for all the yesterdays in your past that got you where you are today. They are in THE PAST. You can't change them, so why punish yourself over them? You CAN change today and tomorrow and all your tomorrows. So, surge ahead!

If today you live a full, healthy day and you promise to do the same tomorrow, I'd say you're on the right track—moving forward. Shape your future, shape yourself. Don't feel sorry for where you've been, only happy about where you're going! Even with each successful day, tomorrow start fresh—it only matters what you're doing now either way!

Supplement your diet with the best the earth can provide!

It's important to ensure that your body is getting all the nutritional supplements and vitamins that you need to sustain your health. I'm not a nutritionist or a doctor, that's why I heed the advice of others in this field. Supplements I believe are necessary in a society where *content* has been compromised. Aside from the more apparent benefits achieved, I've noticed that my hair and nails look healthier than they ever did! Make it a point to be sure your getting all the vitamins and minerals you need.

Eat a few meals, yet less quantity!

Remember the laboratory study where the rats who were fed less lived longer? I think it's safe to say the same is true for us. Keep fruits and vegetables handy at all times. I often feel I'm out grazing in the field, but I am full, satisfied, and trimmed down, so HEY, it must work! If you remember my carrot story, and how I ate so many my teeth were orange, you can follow this example of use a veggie of your own choice. By keeping to fruits and veggies as the highest percent of your intake (next to water, of course), you will look and feel great!

Reward yourself each week for your dedication-with pampering services!

I rewarded myself along the way with things that weren't food related, and you should too. If I had a good week or two, felt good about myself and the strides I had made, I'd reward myself by going to the movies. Once in a while I'd even splurge on some no salt, no butter, popcorn.

Facials, manicures, and pedicures are great rewards, too! There is nothing like being pampered to make you feel special. How about a new CD? Music is great to enhance and change your mood. Don't forget jewelry— for me, this was always nice. I always wanted a thin neck to be able to wear a beautiful gold necklace.

My cosmetic surgery was, of course, what I considered a

very big reward. I didn't do it out of vanity, but feeling it was very much needed. If you think this is something you'd like to consider, start saving now! The time to do it will come before you know it— don't let money be an excuse. Rewarding yourself for achieving any of your goals will keep your commitment strong and increase your self esteem.

> ## Surround yourself with positive, healthy people!

We all have many people in our lives, but not all of them are positive, strong, healthy influences. Now, more than ever, it is important to seek out those who will support your goals and desires. Surround yourself with these people. It's amazing to feel the energy that exists when you're in the presence of others charged with your same positive energy. Even those who have an incredible amount of *being* are sometimes overwhelming— you know, those who just radiate the energy!

Negative people do nothing to keep you motivated and on track. Quite frankly, negative people do not feel comfortable around positive people. They like to talk about negative things. They may be comfortable with the old you— non-threatening, more repressed. BE POSITIVE and you will earn respect, from them and from yourself!

> ## Reject negative thoughts or feelings you have about yourself!

Taking Control of Life!

Every day, every minute, you can consciously make decisions and choices to better yourself. Anything negative is in the past and should remain there. Negativity keeps you down— get pumped up. Each day is a day closer to the new you. Keep telling yourself, "I can do it!"

> **Make a list of all the things you want to do in life. Add to it!**

I function more efficiently if I'm working from a list. Each day I write down everything I need to do, even to pick up the kids ("how could I forget them?"). Doesn't it make sense to write down a TO DO LIST for your life? Maybe you need to go snow skiing, or learn how, or how about a hot air balloon, or, one of my soon to dos— skydiving! Wouldn't that be exciting! Another item on my list is to go to the Academy Awards night! That will be fabulous. When you feel great and healthy, inside and out, nothing is impossible.

> **Set meaningful standards and values for success!**

There are so many ways that you can become successful— NOT just weight loss and lifestyle rejuvenation— how about financial and spiritual? Standards are those guidelines that you personally try to follow— exercising 30 minutes per day; reading 30 minutes per day; praying in the morning and before bed; donating time to a charity, etc. Your values— what is important, what do you value most, second, third,... Put these in writing and you will know from what you base your actions!

Define your primary objective in life to keep your mind focused!

What is your purpose in life? Surely it's NOT to eat and maintain the most unhealthy lifestyle possible? Then, what is it? To be a good parent? To be the best employee? World peace? End world hunger? You can even define your objective on a smaller scale—for the week, the year, or just today! Once you define your purpose, and make it one that motivates you to great things, you'll find that you don't have time to think about food, only making accomplishments!

Develop a daily routine to keep you on your path!

Establish a routine. I once asked a well known motivational speaker/author, Zig Ziglar, on my radio show: how do you maintain your successful life? His answer: "I keep doing the things that I have consistently done." Sticking with what works fosters discipline and constant growth. He is definitely a model for success!

But make a schedule for each day and try to stick to it. Emergencies may arise but those are the exceptions. Keep a general schedule for the day, each about the same, so your mind and body become habitually devoted to what will be the right things! Its easier to accomplish the little tasks one at a time, that will lead to the completion of a larger one!

**Make a list of at least 25
things you enjoy in life!**

Lists, lists, Am I driving you crazy? What's good in your life today? What 25 things can you write down that *you know* are good. Be basic, remember, it's back to the fundamentals in life. For example: people who love you, people you love, a roof over your head, a job that pays money, children, your garden, a talent. The essence is to get your mind back to those things that made us happy as children, when life was full of fun things... because they still are!

**Team up with a partner
who shares your goals!**

The buddy system at its best! You know why this is great? Have you ever seen someone run a marathon by themselves. My guess is not. But I'm sure you've seen or at least heard of the Boston Marathon? Thousands of people run 26 miles to the finish. How do all those people make it?   Training, yes, but not 26 miles at a time. I'm sure that the ability these people have to finish comes from the fact that everyone out there is trying to get to the finish, so each person's motivation helps the next person be motivated to, which helps the next and so on! Now with a partner, you can complete a life's marathon, too!

Begin and maintain a daily exercise program to speed your results!

Exercise, it will increase the speed with which your body recovers to a sound and healthy functioning machine. It will elevate your mood, because it stimulates your body's endorphin and enkephalins (natural pain killers). No one says you have to be a gym dweller. Walking is a refreshing exercise. Even what I call "cheating exercises" where you park your car too far, in order to walk the extra distance when you're parked somewhere. Or taking the stairs instead of the elevator or escalator— a great one! Or power walking through the mall during lunch hour instead of eating...there is so much to see that you will notice you've been missing (window shopping at the same time!).

Remember, each day you are one step closer to achieving your goal!

One day at a time! One step at a time! Every goal in life is this way. Everything takes time and nothing comes easy...unless you break it down into the smallest, most easily achieved parts of the whole. And then in one month you will notice a difference in the way your clothes fit, and the way you feel! Each day builds on the day before. Embrace all the positive tools for success and use them every day. Each morning you'll be one day and one step closer to achieving the new you!

> **Look in the mirror and see the beautiful person inside-that you're letting out!**

You are a beautiful person inside, as seen by the positive attitude you have taken toward life. Let that inner beauty shine through and you will find that all your dreams are within reach. I once read a saying: **If your mind can perceive it, and your heart believes it, then you WILL achieve it.**

> **Don't let anyone steal your dreams!**

Remember the negative people we talked about? People you love can sometimes say things that they don't mean, especially if they don't understand or share your dreams. Don't allow them, or anyone else, to steal your dreams. Have the self-confidence to know that you can do this, that you will do this, and that you will have the body you deserve— no matter what anyone else says.

Make no small dreams, because there is no magic in small dreams. Dream big— *your* dreams belong only to *YOU*! You know what you want in life, what your desires are, the life you want. You can achieve your dreams and, with the help I am giving you and will continue to give you, it will be easier than you think.

> ## Never give up! Make each day a new challenge for success!

Face each new day with excitement and anticipation of good things to come. Challenge yourself daily to succeed in our quest to better your life. Change is never easy. One hundred pounds is not an easy amount of weight to lose. It takes time, effort and determination. You can't give up! If you eat something not healthy for you GET OVER IT! Commit to an extra 10 minutes of walking or treadmill tomorrow (or today!).

> ## Write down all the painful experiences you may have if you don't change.

Let's look at it from the following angles. Give some thought to the negative impact on your life if you don't change! Make this your bottom...your turning point right now!

Physically — Your health, your blood pressure, your back, your life; aren't all these things at risk if you don't change? Is that cake worth dying for? Think of each bad food, each unhealthy bite as one step closer to clogging your arteries completely and causing a heart attack! Now don't those foods sound disgusting at the expense of what they do!?

Socially — If you're even close to the size that I was, try going to a modern movie theater. I thought I'd never get out of the seat once I jammed my rear end and thighs in. Even now, at a size 6, those seats still feel pretty small—just who did they have in mind when they designed them, Twiggy? It's the same on buses, trains, airlines—and try going through a turnstile...EMBARRASSING! Do you have the energy to join your kids in kite flying? Do you feel self-conscious at an office party? Do you want to go roller or ice skating or snow skiing but can't?

Financially — Many studies have shown that heavy people frequently are not treated fairly at work. They are often passed over for promotions, raises, bonuses, etc. I do not agree nor condone any behavior that treats people unfairly, but it does exist. Are you satisfied with your financial situation? Do you want to improve it? Once you are practicing a healthy lifestyle, you will be amazed at all the opportunities that present themselves.

> ## Have faith in yourself and each action you take!

You must have faith that God has given you the ability to accomplish anything you set your heart and mind to. God helps those who help themselves! Somewhere inside, you will find the strength that you need to succeed. Believe in yourself! You may have heard: *"If your mind perceives it, and your heart believes it, then you can achieve it!"*

> ## Remember, your dreams and goals are always within reach!

Each day I tell my husband, Patrick, how happy I am that we are on a journey toward accomplishing great things, and having a positive impact on the world. The positive energy we both have, collectively allows us ten times the amount of energy that we would have individually.

A great inventor, Thomas Edison, apparently tried over 2,000 experiments before inventing the light bulb. Two-thousand failures? NO. He claimed they were 2,000 learning experiences. Remember this: **A successful person gets up one more time than a failing one.** What if he had stopped after 1,999 tries. Your dreams are only one step away!!

In Closing

Dr. White often remarks on how energetic and full of life I am. I find it both amazing and sad that for so many years I wasn't like this. At times during the writing, I shed a tear thinking about the misery I was in, and how happy I am now that I made the decision to turn around. I want you to do that to. As he told me "Taking control of your life is never easy." That may be true, however, taking one small step at a time will lead you miles ahead in just a matter of weeks!

I sincerely hope that you've enjoyed reading my story. I truly believe that I've given you the tools to begin building a solid foundation for creating your new body and new life!

From today on, your choices in life are going to be based on what is best for you. Not on another diet. Although you may see thin people eating junk food, and ask yourself why you can't have that and be thin, don't! Thin or not it is still junk food, and making a junk body out of a healthy one.

Put yourself, your dignity, and your pride first from now on! Don't let anyone stand in your way, especially yourself—your mental blocks. Wake up and say each day... "I'm in charge here!" Think about doing only one action for getting healthy each day, and working up to several. Starting with the first good meal. Just one. When you get by that and its time to eat again, think only about that one meal—one good, healthy meal. Continue this and build on it, two days from now, add a short workout/exercise. In three weeks, you'll have your habits down. Remember: it takes 21 days to develop a new habit. Twenty-one days! That's not long at all to get into the habit of your new healthy lifestyle! I've read somewhere an interesting point to keep in mind: People who were very near death were surveyed as to what they would have changed about their lives if they could. The results showed that **nearly all surveyed regretted NOT doing something** rather than regretted something they had done! Don't miss your opportunity to do what you need, want, and are fully capable of!!

It's your turn to go out and conquer the world. Go for it! For yourself. If you ever struggle or have a success story, no matter how big or small, please contact me and let me know! I would love to hear from you. It always helps to know there are people out there who are changing their lives for the better!! Write or e-mail using either method below, and I will answer to try and help.

In good health,

Julia
God bless you!

To e-mail go to: **www.JuliaHavey.com**

or write to: **Julia Havey**
                P.O. Box 6794
                St. Louis, MO 63144-6794

GROCERY

LIST

&

RECIPES

Grocery List

Keep it simple, start with the basics. Obviously, you don't need to buy everything on this list every time you shop. I recommend having these around as often as possible!

Always get a low-fat variety of any item if possible.

Staples:

garlic pepper
lemon pepper
beef bouillon
soy sauce
pickle relish
celery salt
pasta sauce
wheat flour
mayonnaise

cilantro
mint
pumpkin spice
salad dressing(s)
paprika
dry mustard
basil
oregano
parsley

Fruits:

apples	oranges	bananas
grapes	raspberries	peaches
honeydew	strawberries	mango
watermelon	blueberries	cantaloupe

..........eat a lot of fruit!!!

Make sure that you only buy enough to eat for the next few days, you don't want to over stock and have it go bad and waste money! Shop smart!

Vegetables

asparagus	snow peas	broccoli
mushrooms	red peppers	avocado
yellow peppers	corn cobs	potatoes
green peppers	cabbage	carrots
celery purple	mini carrots	zucchini
green beans	yellow squash	spaghetti squash
bib lettuce	sprouts	spinach
romaine lettuce	tomatoes	cucumber
onions	beans-all types that you like	

Bottled Water:
As much as you can afford and as much as you can drink! If you're drinking out of the tap, I recommend getting a filter.

Starches:

multi grain bagels	multi grain breads
low fat bran muffins	pasts, pita bread,
flour tortilla shells,	oatmeal, bran cereals
cream of wheat	brown rice
Gardenburgers (meatless patties)- all varieties,	

Remember the pyramid: keep starches to a minimum!

Meats and Proteins

low-fat cottage cheese	low/non-fat yogurt
skim milk	Lean ground sirloin
low fat cheeses	beef tenderloin
pork tenderloin	turkey breast
eggs	Gardenburgers tofu

fish—all types (lighter colored the healthiest)
chicken breast-boneless, skinless
beans and lentils

RECIPES

I consistently ate these things during my 130 lb. weight loss:

Veggie Sandwich

2 slices nine-grain bread (keep frozen until needed)
     2 slices red pepper
     2 slices green pepper
     2 slices tomato
     1 slice low-fat Lorraine Swiss
     broccoli slaw*

Stack ingredients between 2 slices of bread. Microwave on HIGH approximately 2 minutes. (Or broil in conventional oven approximately 1 minute on each side).

*broccoli slaw - obtain from your supermarket in packaged, prepared form. If unavailable, make your own by shredding broccoli, carrots and purple cabbage and mixing together.

Best Brown Rice

1 cup brown rice
1 Tbsp beef or chicken bullion
Cook rice according to package directions, adding bullion to flavor the water. When cooked add: 2 Tbsp low-fat condensed cream of mushroom soup. Mix well and serve.

Low-Fat Pasta

2 cups cooked rigatoni noodles
½ cup each: green beans, baby carrots, sliced zucchini, yellow squash, white onion, sliced tomato
Mix together in a bowl and toss with: ¼ cup olive oil
¼ cup cider vinegar and Grey Poupon™ mustard
May be eaten warm or cold.

Bean Salad
Mix together ½ cup each:
red beans, pinto beans, black beans
and navy beans
Add: ½ cup finely chopped onion
2 Tbsp non-fat mayonnaise
2 Tbsp bread and butter pickle juice
Chill several hours or overnight. Enjoy.!

Veggie Pizza
1 ready-to-cook 8" pizza crust
½ cup each: diced tomatoes, red pepper, green pepper,
red onion, yellow squash, zucchini
broccoli, cauliflower
Brush pizza crust with olive oil and top with vegetables
Sprinkle lightly with: shredded mozzarella cheese,
fat-free Romano or Parmesan cheese
Microwave on HIGH approximately 5 to 8 minutes or bake
in conventional oven at 400° for approximately 20 minutes.

Veggie Pasta
1 cup cooked spaghetti noodles
½ cup each: broccoli, cauliflower, carrots,
corn niblets and celery (substitute, add,
or remove any vegetables you wish)

Place ingredients in a microwave-safe bowl and mix together. Toss in: 2 Tbsp fat free margarine. Sprinkle with fat-fee Parmesan cheese and place lid on bowl, but do not seal. Microwave on HIGH approximately 2 to 3 minutes until noodles are hot and vegetables are slightly crisp. Mix well. Serve.

Note: with the pasta and potato recipes, serve moderate portions.

Twice Baked Potato
1 large potato
¼ cup plain non-fat yogurt
1 tsp non-fat cream cheese, at room temperature
dash prepared horseradish
1 Tbsp green onions
1 tsp chopped fresh parsley
a pinch of paprika

Preheat oven to 350º. Bake potato 1 hour or until done. When cool enough to handle, slice in half lengthwise and spoon out pulp into a bowl, reserving shells. Add remaining ingredients except the shells and paprika. Spoon mixture into shells and sprinkle with paprika. Bake 10 minutes or until heated through.

Red Beans and Rice
1 package red beans and rice
2 cans diced tomatoes, drained
1 tsp chili powder (or to taste)

Prepare red beans and rice according to package directions.
Add tomatoes and chili powder 5 minutes before cooking time ends.

(This recipe makes approximately 6 servings at 200 calories per serving with 0 grams of fat. It is very filling and nutritious, freezes well for serving at a later day.)

CAESAR GOURMET

1 Gardenburger Savory Mushroom veggie patty
2 Slices whole grain sourdough bread
¼ cup chopped romaine lettuce
2 slices red onion/and or tomato
1Tbsp freshly grated Parmesan cheese
2 Tbsp Fat free Caesar dressing
Olive oil spray, ground pepper

Toast bread. Spray pan with oil, saute patty and onion till golden. Stack bun with all ingredients, top with bun. Serve warm.

SICILIAN PARMESAN

1 Fire Roasted Gardenburger patty
1 whole grain Focaccia bread slice, split in two
⅓ cup Marinara sauce
1 Tbsp fresh parmesan cheese
1 Yellow zucchini squash, sliced diagonally
fresh basil, olive oil spray

Saute patty and squash in oil till golden. Place atop focaccia, top with heated marinara, basil and cheese.

I recently read a story of a 400lb. woman who fought her insurance company until they agreed to pay for her to have her stomach stapled shut so that she could lose weight.

After the surgery, and 50lbs. thinner she remarks, "this surgery is the best thing that ever happened to me,...before it, I could eat a whole box of Poptarts and not feel full."

This is so typical of the obesity problem— it is not that her stomach needed to be stapled— she needed to refrain from overeating!